Keto Diet Cookbook For Women After 50

The Step-By-Step Guide for Senior Women to Approach Ketogenic Diet, Hot to Regain Metabolism and Balance Hormones in 30-Day with 90 Delicious Recipes

Claudia Giordano

Table of Contents

INTRODUCTION

Although I'm 52 years old, I'm in the best (and hottest!) shape of my life. The kind of hot that makes you want to pinch yourself to validate if what you're experiencing is truly real life. I don't count calories. I dip my bacon in mayonnaise and snack on jars of almond butter with zero guilt.

Thanks to the keto diet, my body has found its happy place. Weight loss is effortless—I've lost twenty pounds in two months! My skin is glowing, and I'm not a slave to pack-along snacks, cravings, or energy lulls anymore.

The secret? Switching into a state of nutritional ketosis, where the body goes from burning glucose as energy to burning fat as energy. In nutritional ketosis, the body becomes a fat-burning machine, effectively breaking down fatty acids into ketone bodies that are used, even by the brain, as fuel. And we do this by following an eating style of high-fat, low carbs, and moderate protein, also known as **"keto"** or **"ketogenic."**

In this book, we focus on benefiting the body long term, through paleo-friendly strategies packed with whole foods and rich nutrition that are optimal for women **over 50.**

Keep in mind that right around the age of 50, our bodies start going through quite a bit of change, including:

- Menopause
- Enlargement of the heart (high blood pressure can weaken the cardiac muscles)
- Skin becomes tough and dry

- The production of collagen (this repairs skin and hair) slows down
- Osteoporosis

All of us over-50 women can make good use of this diet and lifestyle to keep us fit, active, and free from all the ailments that are linked with this age. Keep reading to find out how!

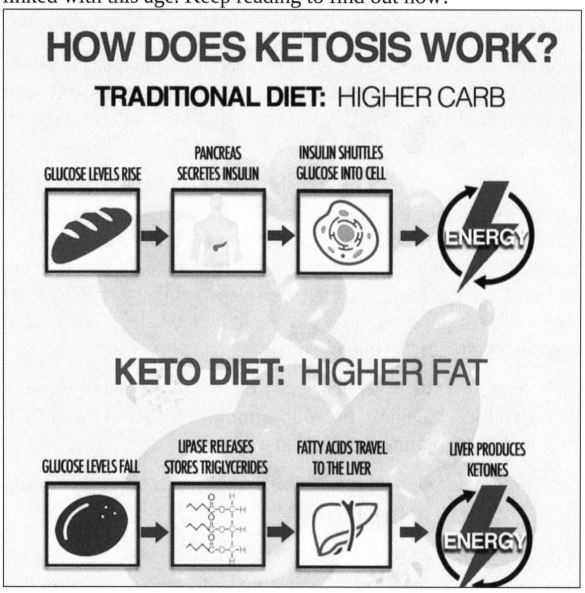

Important tips for the keto diet after 50

A las, as us women get older, keeping off those pesky extra pounds gets harder, doesn't it?

If this is happening to you, you are not alone. Over 40 million women in the US, 13 million in the UK, and many more millions around the world are estimated to be going through menopause, which usually occurs between ages 49 and 52.

Weight gain is very common during this transition, no matter what diet you are eating.

Here are some very important tips to help you use the keto diet properly

1. Get the right amount of protein

As a whole, the advice from me is to eat between 1.2 to 1.7 grams of protein per kilogram of reference body weight per day. Reference body weight is the halfway point of what is considered healthy (not to be confused with ideal body weight), so a woman whose reference body weight is 70 kg (154 lbs) should aim for 70 to 119 grams of protein per day.

Just remember: Protein intake can be a balancing act. Too little protein over the long run, especially as we age, can lead to poor muscle growth and frailty.

2. Don't eat too much fat

Once you're fat-adapted, it's important to avoid consuming excess fat.

Speaking from experience, one of the great joys of low-carb keto eating is including fat at every meal after years of avoiding it.

However, experts note that a keto diet is not carte blanche to gorge yourself on fat. If you want to lose weight, you have to burn your fat stores for energy rather than consuming all the energy you need by eating fat. So if you're struggling to lose weight, stop the bulletproof coffee and fat bombs for now.

3. Try intermittent fasting

After becoming fat-adapted, you may find that your hunger pangs diminish, making it easy to go for longer periods without eating.

Many people naturally stop eating breakfast—they just aren't hungry when they wake up. The number one rule of low-carb eating is to eat when you are hungry and stop when you are full. So if you are not hungry, try intermittent fasting (IF).

Start by skipping breakfast and just eating lunch and dinner within an eight-hour window, which is called a 16:8 fast. Or you can try eating dinner one night, then fasting until dinner the next night, which is known as a 24-hour fast.

When people are doing low-carb keto eating, they are often not hungry for 16 or 24 hours. Such fasts are safe and healthy, as long as you have some weight to lose.

However, avoid fasting if you are underweight. Eat when you are hungry, don't eat when you are not, and stop when you are full.

4. Cut out alcohol

Many people love the fact that on a low carb or keto diet, they can have a glass of dry wine from time to time. However, if you are experiencing a weight-loss plateau or gaining weight, cut out all alcohol for now until weight loss starts again. Even a few drinks a week might cause a stall.

5. Get enough sleep

During menopause, many women find their quality of sleep sharply deteriorates, often because of hot flashes and night sweats.

Tips for better sleep include:

1. Sleep in a cool, dark room.
2. Wear earplugs and eyeshades.
3. Limit screen time and blue light before bed (or try the glasses that block blue light).
4. Go to bed and get up at the same time each day.
5. Stop drinking coffee by noon and limit caffeine consumption in all forms.
6. Avoid alcohol before bed.
7. Get exposure to natural daylight each day.

6. Be realistic

- Realistic expectations are particularly important for women of all ages.

- Some of us are aiming for an arbitrary number on a scale, perhaps from a long time ago or an idealized weight we have never achieved—a number that has no real bearing or relationship to our actual health and wellness.

- Measure your success by a loss of inches, rather than the scale.

Remember that yo u ' re in this for the long haul. I t ' s an investment in your health as you get older. Have patience! Your long-term goal is to make a permanent lifestyle change as well as lose the excess fat.

MY INTENTION

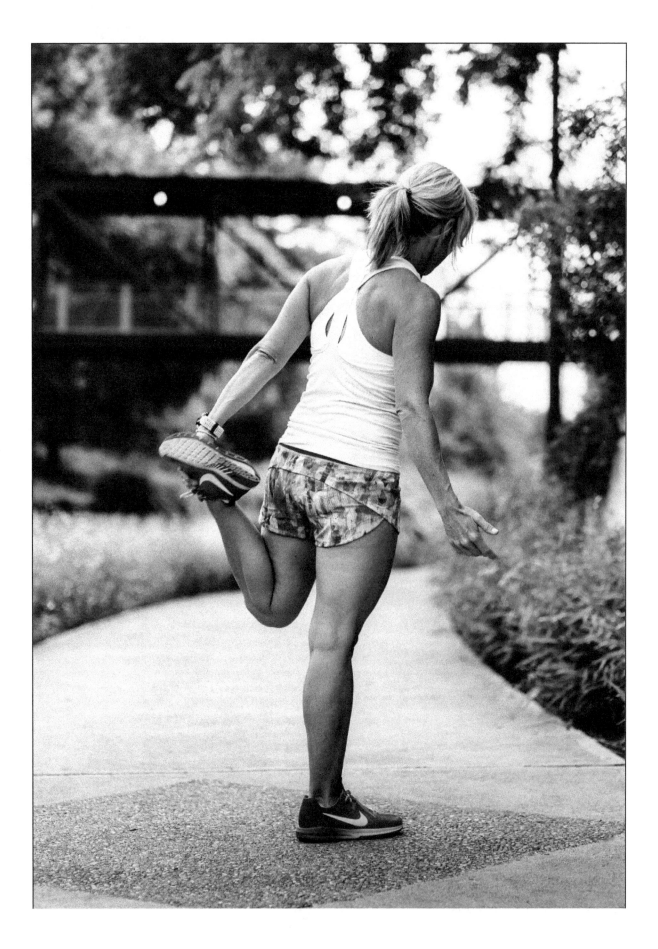

This book is meant to highlight how easy and effortless living a dairy-free keto life can be.

You may be thinking, but she has only been on this for two months, how could she possibly know that this lifestyle can be a lifelong ticket to lasting health? Great question!

My answer, in short, is because everything in this Book is intended to counteract the issues that get in the way of lifelong health, especially blood sugar.

I've experienced more life-altering positive changes with this next evolution in my eating style than I have with any other pattern. It's the easiest, most effortless, and most rewarding approach I've ever experimented with. A double bonus: The medical studies and research I've read points to blood sugar regulation through a high fat, low-carb diet being the ticket to lasting health. I have no doubt that the two months I've spent exploring this whole food-based ketogenic eating style has brought me closer to a life filled with endless happy, healthy days than any other approach I've tried in the past. It truly is an evolution!

Coupled with my whole foods-loving approach, this Book satisfies all of the markers necessary for lifelong health—the natural reduction in calories, boosted saturated fats, blood sugar control, boosted cell health, ample mitochondria action, and more.

There aren't a lot of "recipes" in the meal plan, as this is an introduction to nutritional ketosis. When I was first getting started, I realized that I had no idea what 75% fat, 10% carbs, and 15% protein looked like on a plate, let alone what it felt like in my body. So I'm going to break it down for you!

CHAPTER ONE

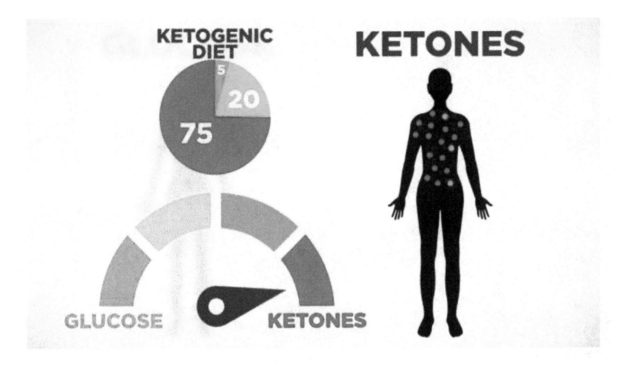

The Keto Basics

Though not mandatory (you can skip over this part if you don't care to know how this all works), understanding how the body functions and fully knowing what's at play here makes following the ketogenic lifestyle more meaningful. At least, it does for me.

To really understand what's going on here, we have to start from the very beginning, and the digestive system is the very best place to start.

The Digestive Process

When we consume foo d …

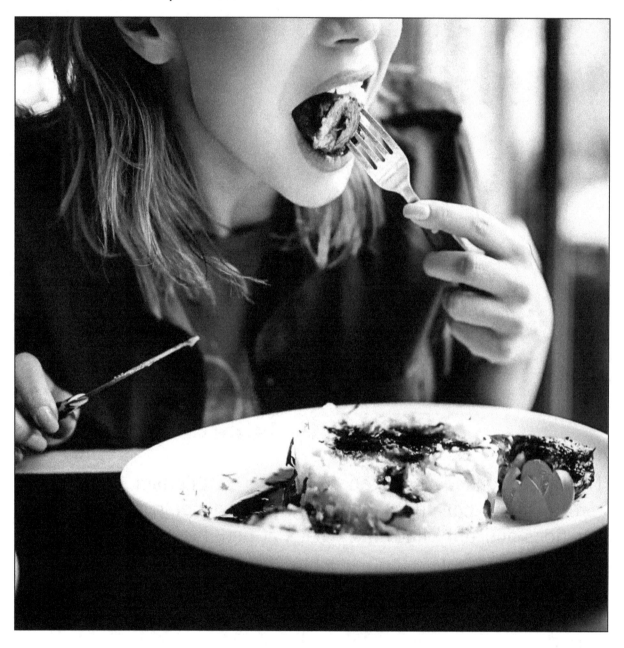

1. The site of initial carbohydrate breakdown occurs in the mouth. Your teeth and tongue take the first steps in battering food into bits. As they are shredding and grinding, more saliva is squirted into the food to moisten and soften it. The saliva contains chemicals called enzymes, which break down the carbohydrates in food (this enzyme release triggers insulin to start prepping for action).

2. When you have finished chewing, you swallow; the mouthful of food makes its way down the esophagus to the stomach. Food does not free-fall down to the stomach but is squeezed along by the muscles in the esophagus. This squeezing/pushing action by the muscles is called peristalsis (perry-STAL-sis).

3. The site of initial protein breakdown occurs in the stomach, where food is treated to a strong acid bath as it's churned around by the stomach's muscular walls. These walls are protected by a mucus lining, which shields the stomach from its own gastric juices (made up of pepsin enzyme and acids).

4. Up until now, carbohydrates have been broken down slightly in the mouth, and proteins have been broken down slightly in the stomach. Fats have not had their turn.

5. Now, for the breakdown of fats and further breakdown of carbohydrates and proteins. Food is now a mashed-up milky liquid, thanks to the stomach. It enters the

duodenum (the beginning of the small intestine), where it is treated with a round of enzymes and bile to break the carbohydrates, proteins, and fats down even further.

6. From there, the substance enters the small intestine—a twenty-foot-long, curly tube with a shaggy lining. The walls of the small intestine are lined with millions of tiny finger-like projections called villi. The villi absorb the usable parts of the broken-down food into the bloodstream.

7. The non-useful parts of the food continue to move into the large intestine, which absorbs some of the water and salt. The remainder of the material is compacted and then sent out the anus as solid waste or feces.

Carbohydrate Digestion

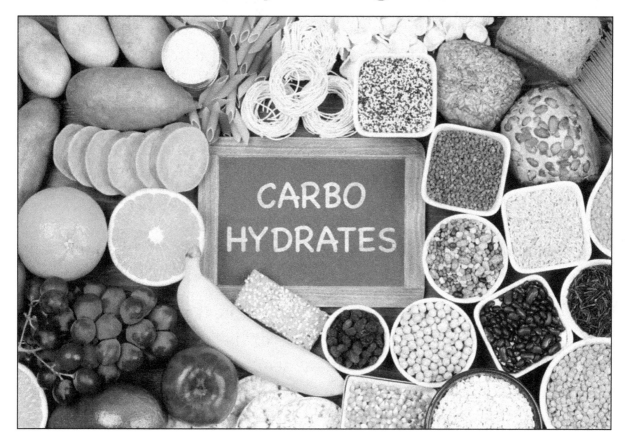

Carbs are organic molecules that are made up of carbon, hydrogen, and oxygen. There are three principal carbohydrates present in foods…

1. Simple Sugars (aka simple carbohydrates)

2. Polysaccharides (aka complex carbohydrates)

3. Fiber

Simple Sugars (aka simple carbohydrates) have three classifications, and several sub-segments below each class. It's a web of sugary confusion! The simplest of simple sugars are glucose, fructose, and galactose. These are called monosaccharides

—this is how all sugars end up in our body when all is said and done.

For instance, if you consume white sugar (sucrose), the body will break it down into glucose and fructose. If you consume a glass of milk (lactose), the body will break it down into galactose and glucose.

Then there are oligosaccharides—simple sugars that consist of several sugars bound together. These unique carbohydrates cannot be easily digested by our regular digestive path and have to go to the large intestine to be eaten up by the bacteria there. Examples of oligosaccharide foods are onions, asparagus, garlic, banana, and chives.

Polysaccharides (aka complex carbohydrates) undergo substantial digestion before being absorbed. Starch is a polysaccharide—the main carbohydrate source for plant seeds and vegetables grown in the ground. Think potatoes, corn, rice, pasta, and cereal. Starches are broken down into glucose by the body.

Another polysaccharide is cellulose, a carbohydrate that is indigestible in the body, adding bulk to the stool.

Fiber is another form of carbohydrate, one that is present in many polysaccharides. Fiber's main purpose is to aid in elimination.

The body converts digestible carbohydrates (the parts of the carbohydrate that are non-fiberous) into glucose, which our cells use as fuel. Some carbs (simple sugars, aka simple carbohydrates) break down quickly into glucose while others (polysaccharides, aka complex carbohydrates) are slowly broken down and enter the bloodstream more gradually.

The major takeaway here is that ALL dietary forms of carbohydrates are made up of sugar (glucose). Sweet potato, white bread, whole grains, candy, potato chips, fruit, kale—all contain components that become sugar in the body. So that you fully "get the picture" on this carbohydrate thing, perhaps it would be helpful for me to list some sources of carbohydrates, yes?

Okay, here goes…

Bagels, bread, stuffing, buns, croutons, pancakes, English muffins, pita bread, tortillas, corn, waffles, wraps, beans, oatmeal, cornmeal, lentils, flour, hummus, rice, quinoa, pasta, peas, potatoes, squash, sweet potato, cow's milk, rice milk, soy milk, yogurt, apples, cantaloupe, banana, apricots, dates, grapefruit, prunes, raspberries, watermelon, carrot juice, apple juice, tomato juice, cranberry juice, kiwi, alcohol, biscuits, cookies, donuts, muffins, fruit pie, cupcakes, chocolate, potato chips, pretzels, crackers, sherbet, ice cream, tortilla chips, Jell-O, granola, cereal, French fries, apple butter, barbecue sauce, oats, cranberry sauce, salad dressing, ketchup, jams, jellies, candies, mints, gum, soda, gravy, honey mustard, dipping sauces, plum sauce, hollandaise sauce, maple syrup, honey, agave nectar, coconut sugar, coconut nectar, noodles, lasagna, egg rolls, cream soups, soups, chutney, arrowroot, tapioca, chickpea flour, sorghum, millet, amaranth, muesli, shredded wheat, popcorn, rice cakes, pudding, custard, almonds, cashews, pumpkin seeds, gar- banzo beans, lima beans, green peas, carrots, pinto beans, navy beans, beets, onions, parsnips, bell peppers, spinach, greens, turnips, yams, white sugar, dates, date sugar, dried fruit, flour, pizz a .

The key here is that, regardless of if you are consuming a simple or complex carbohydrate, it will turn into "sugar" in the body.

Introduction to a New Way

The "Healthy" High-Carb Approach

Our current high-carbohydrate eating style of whole grains, several servings of fruits and vegetables, and minimal intake of fats have been touted as "healthy." Now you know from the previous section that all forms of carbohydrate—fruits, vegetables, grains, sugars, and anything starchy—are primarily broken down into glucose and stored in your body as glycogen.

When you have more glycogen than what's needed for immediate energy, your body will store excess in the liver, then the muscles, and if everything is full, the excess is converted into triglycerides and stored in your blood. Psst...this is *not* a good thing!

Relying on carbohydrates for fuel is:

- Not sustainable; we can only store a couple thousand calories of carbohydrates at any given time.
- Preventing us from getting a handle on our blood sugar, causing endless cravings, various daily eating times, and weight gain.
- Leading to triglycerides being stored in the blood, the major risk factor to heart disease.
- Slowly killing us.

What is the Keto Diet?

What is the ketogenic diet exactly? The classic ketogenic diet is a very low-carb diet plan that was originally designed in the 1920s for patients with epilepsy by researchers working at Johns Hopkins Medical Center. Researchers found that fasting—avoiding consumption of all foods for a brief period of time (such as with intermittent fasting), including those that provide carbohydrates—helped reduce the amount of seizures patients suffered, in addition to having other positive effects on body fat, blood sugar, cholesterol, and hunger levels.

Unfortunately, long-term fasting is not a feasible option for more than a few days, therefore the keto diet was developed to mimic the same beneficial effects of fasting.

Essentially, the keto diet for beginners works by "tricking" the body into acting as if it's fasting (while reaping intermittent fasting benefits) through a strict elimination of glucose that is found in carbohydrate foods. Today, the standard keto diet goes by several different names including the "low-carbohydrate" or "very-low-carbohydrate ketogenic diet."

Keto Diet Fat Burner vs. Sugar Burner

At the core of the classic keto diet is severely restricting intake of all or most foods with sugar and starch (carbohydrates). These foods are broken down into sugar (insulin and glucose) in our blood once we eat them, and if these levels become too high, extra calories are much more easily stored as body fat and result in unwanted weight gain. However, when glucose levels are cut off due to low-carb intake, the body starts to burn fat instead and produces ketones that can be measured in the blood (using urine strips, for example).

Keto diets, like most low-carb diets, work through the elimination of glucose. Because most folks live on a high-carb diet, our bodies normally run on glucose (or sugar) for energy. We cannot make glucose and only have about twenty-four hours' worth stored in our muscle tissue and liver. Once glucose is no longer available from food sources, we begin to burn stored fat instead, or fat from our food.

Therefore, when you're following a ketogenic diet plan for beginners, your body is burning fat for energy rather than carbohydrates, so in the process, most people lose weight and excess body fat rapidly, even when consuming lots of fat and adequate calories through their daily food intake. Another major benefit of the keto diet is that there's no need to count calories, feel hungry, or attempt to burn loads of calories through hours of intense exercise.

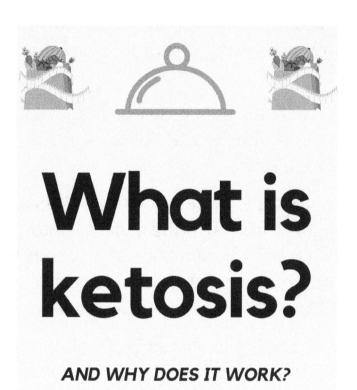

AND WHY DOES IT WORK?

<u>What is Ketosis?</u>

Nutritional ketosis is a state where your body is "deprived" of glucose; achieved when carbohydrate intake is decreased, and protein intake is moderated. In this state, you switch to using fat as energy instead of carbohydrates. This process—of using fat as fuel —produces ketone bodies that are converted into substrates for the Krebs Cycle (energy production). Once you're in nutritional ketosis, the storage of triglycerides in blood no longer applies. Blood sugar and insulin levels are reduced, levels of HDL cholesterol increase, and the visceral fats around your vital organs are "eaten up" as fuel.

In nutritional ketosis, we're tripping the metabolic switch, leading to so much more than just weight loss.

The Keto Beginning is about finding our body's happy place and using fatty acids and the generation of ketone bodies as a reliable fuel for constant, steady energy. The brain, the heart, our hormones, and every cell in the body loves ketones.

Ketones are a highly renewable energy source that our major organs use effortlessly to promote lasting health in a blood sugar-balanced environment.

This is nutritional ketosis, not to be confused with diabetic ketoacidosis—a dangerous condition where ketones spike and blood sugar increases to alarming rates.

This occurs primarily in diabetes type 1 (and sometimes 2) patients who are not receiving enough insulin to bring glucose into their cells. Regardless of how low carbohydrate intake is, a person with a normal pancreas cannot enter diabetic ketoacidosis because even a trace amount of insulin will keep ketone levels at a safe level.

Having said that, three groups of people should NOT play around with nutritional ketosis unless under the care of a professional in a one-on-one setting—pregnant women, diabetics (type 1), and individuals with kidney disease or a kidney imbalance.

Clarification of "Being in Ketosis" and "Being Keto-Adapted"

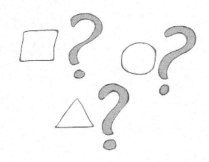

CLARIFICATION Our bodies burn whatever fuel for energy that is available—glucose, fatty acids, ketones, alcohol, etc.

Following a ketogenic eating style puts you into a state of ketosis. What this means is that your body is breaking down enough fat so that there are ketones in your bloodstream. This happens either by fasting or with the support of a low-carb, high-fat, moderate-protein eating style. Being "in ketosis" is a normal metabolic state.

One of the goals of the ketogenic eating style is becoming "keto-adapted." Being keto-adapted means that your body is primed for functioning with very little glucose. This is the END goal of the Keto Beginning.

When you first enter ketosis (a result of following a ketogenic eating style for a couple of days), you are using fat for energy, but it's in limited amounts at first because you don't have as many fat-converting enzymes in your body. Different enzymes are involved in breaking down fat than breaking down glucose. And, up until now, you've been breaking down excess glucose more so than fats, so it takes the body a bit of time to "catch up" and store these enzymes when you first get started. This is one of the reasons many people feel tired at the beginning of following a ketogenic eating style. Once the enzymes are built up, your cells change the way they acquire energy and you become fully keto-adapted.

The process of becoming keto-adapted can take a few weeks to a month, depending on the person. Once you're keto-adapted, fatty acids and their substrates, ketone bodies, become your body's preferred fuel. Hormone levels change, the energy stores in the liver and muscle (glycogen) are depleted, your body carries around less water, and your energy is boosted to normal levels again.

This is why this Book outlines sticking with the plan for thirty days before deviation, so that one can become fully keto-adapted.

When the body is keto-adapted and gets an overdose of carbohydrates, the process of getting back into ketosis doesn't take as long as the initial keto adaptation because the body is primed to use fat as energy. When too many carbohydrates are consumed, the carbohydrates (glucose) still takes precedence over fat for fuel because excess blood sugar is fatal and so your body needs to handle the sugar first.

When the overdose occurs, a couple of things happen: glycogen (the way glucose is stored in the liver and muscles) gets replenished, leading to water retention, insulin rises, and hormone levels are boosted. While this is occurring, you are not burning ketones. Once the glucose is depleted, the body will go back into ketosis.

As you begin your keto journey, the more often you have sugar (or, an abundance of carbohydrates past what your body can manage on a daily basis without spiking insulin release), the longer it takes to become keto-adapted.

Your Goal for this BOOK

Become keto-adapted! This simply means that your body becomes efficient at being able to burn fat, and functions very well even in the presence of very little glucose.

By becoming keto-adapted, your body literally will become a fat-burning machine!

Chapter Two

Following Keto

What to Eat on a Keto Diet?

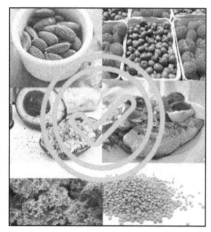

When it comes to keto food choices, choosing nutrient-dense foods is key to maintaining good health—it's not all bacon and butter! What you eat matters and can directly affect your overall health, well-being, and how successful you are on any type of diet.

Foods that fit into a keto diet are typically high-fat low-carb foods and non-starchy veggies. Protein sources can also be included. Here is a rough list of the most nutritious foods that fit into a keto meal plan.

Healthy Keto Fats

- **Nuts and nut butters made without added sugar**
- **Seeds**
- **Plant-based oils**
- **Avocado**
- **Olives**

- **Cacao**

Low-Carb Fruits and Vegetables

- **Non-starchy veggies: leafy greens, radishes, cauliflower, broccoli, tomato, eggplant, zucchini, cucumber, peppers, green beans, celery, bok choy, jicama, mushrooms, artichokes, cabbage, beets, onions, and carrots.**
- **Melon and strawberries (one serving provides half of the recommended 20 grams of carbs).**
- **All fresh herbs**

Keto Proteins

- **Eggs**
- **Fatty fish like salmon, mackerel, and herring**
- **Bison, beef, pork, goat, and lamb**
- **Chicken with skin**
- **Shellfish**
- **Cottage cheese, cheese, and unsweetened yogurt**
- **Organ meats**

Keto Sweeteners

- **Erythritol**
- **Monk Fruit**
- **Stevia**
- **Other artificial sweeteners**

What Foods to Avoid?

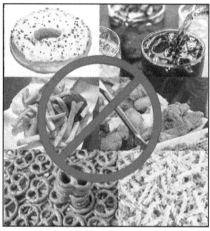 Since a keto meal plan is all about hitting your macros, just about any food can fit into this eating plan except carb-containing foods. Many carb sources will put you over your daily limit in a single serving or less. Here are some of the top foods/types of foods that you'll want to avoid on a keto diet.

High-Carb Foods

- **All grains, pastas, and breads**
- **Beans, lentils, and other legumes**
- **Corn**
- **Potatoes**
- **Most fruits and dried fruits**
- **Juice and soda**
- **Milk**
- **Desserts**
- **Breaded meats and other breaded fried foods**
- **Sugars: maple, honey, agave, table sugar, etc.**

Keto Beverages

Many beverages are loaded with added sugar or made from juice blends that are naturally higher in carbs. When looking for drinks that fit into a keto plan, it's always best to check the nutrition facts label.

Keto Drinks

- **Water**
- **Sparkling water/club soda**
- **Tea and coffee, unsweetened**
- **Flavored water with no added sugar**
- **Wheatgrass or other green vegetable juices made without fruit**
- **Artificially sweetened beverages**

Low-Carb Alcohol

- **Clear liquor: vodka, gin, rum**
- **Scotch and bourbon**
- **Light beers**
- **Champagne and some wine**

Personalize Your Plan & Calculate Your Macros

Working closely with a keto-specialized dietitian and personal chef for this guide, we've put together a plan that provides a great framework for you.

As I mentioned earlier, each person is different and may require specific tweaks to get into ketosis. Some people can metabolize carbs more quickly and can consume more than 60 grams of carbs per day and stay in ketosis. More likely, however, you may even need to stay under 50 grams to get into ketosis.

The only true way to find out if your body is in ketosis or not is to test. However, you can choose to customize this plan based on your own personal needs like energy expenditure, personal weight loss or weight-gain goals, etc.

For this challenge, we went with approximately:

- **15% Nutrient-Dense Carbohydrates**
- **25% High-Quality Protein**
- **60% Healthy Fats**

If you'd like to personalize your macronutrients, here's a GREAT calculator online that will help you figure out your specific percentages in more detail:

http://keto-calculator.ankerl.com/

You'll need your body fat percentage to complete the calculation. When you stop in for measurements, we will provide you with this number.

If you do end up adjusting the percentages, you'll have to make the appropriate changes in the recipes as well, as they are currently structured for the 15/25/60 ratio.

Avoiding the Keto Flu

In the beginning, some people experience the "keto flu" when they are transitioning into ketosis. Many people who begin the ketosis process for the first time get flu-like symptoms, feel like all their energy is drained, and basically just feel awful.

I'm going to teach you EXACTLY how to avoid it. Most people do this WRONG, so please make sure to follow these guidelines!

The primary reason people get keto flu is because their electrolytes get out of balance.

1. **Drink a LOT of water.** You need to be drinking at LEAST half your body weight in ounces per day.

2. **Use Pink Himalayan Rock Salt.** About 1 tsp. per day should do the trick. A simple trick is to put 1 tsp. of pink sea salt in a bowl on the counter. By the end of the day, make sure you have used up the entire teaspoon. Himalayan salt has more minerals and trace elements than other salts. It's also a very pure and unprocessed product. Sodium is an important electrolyte, so this is the perfect way to get high-quality salt in your diet (stay far away from white table salt)!

3. **CALM.** This is one of my favorite supplements. Magnesium not only helps combat stress in the body, but

it's an important mineral that's required for more than 700 biochemical reactions in your body.

4. **Homemade Bone Broth.** This will help balance the vitamins and minerals in your body in the most incredible way. Broth is amazing for healing and promoting a healthy digestive tract, reducing joint pain and inflammation, and promoting hair and nail growth (and some say it can help with cellulite because it helps maintain the integrity of the cell walls!).

Additional Supplements

In addition to the supplements listed above for avoiding the keto flu, I recommend taking the following supplements. These are optional and not required.

1.
MCT Oil – This will help you to get into ketosis faster. MCT stands for Medium-Chain Triglycerides. It's basically a refined version of coconut oil that is 6x more potent.

Start with 1 tsp. and build from there up to 1 tbsp. I usually add 1 tbsp. (with some grass-fed butter) in the morning to my bulletproof coffee! You'll love what it does for your mental clarity.

You can get MCT oil at health food stores, nutritional supplement stores, online, and even at some well-stocked grocery stores.

2.
Probiotics – Did you know that up to 70% of your immune system resides in your gut? Probiotics can help restore balance

back to your digestive system and provide an overall boost to your immune system.

The bacteria in your body outnumber your cells by more than 10 to 1. Remember, the good bacteria help to keep you in check. They help to fight against the "bad" bacteria, viruses, and other pathogens.

It's really important to give this good bacteria an extra hand because the toxins, chemicals, and any antibiotics we are exposed to will kill off these microscopic warriors.

3.

Omega 3s (Fish Oil) – Omega 3s help reduce inflammation in the body, increase your ability to burn fat, strengthen your immune system, improve circulation, improve good cholesterol, and the list goes on and on.

4.

Rhodiola – If you live a high-stress life, rhodiola can help combat some of the effects. It helps fight fatigue, boosts memory, and increase work capacity to improve productivity.

Testing Your Personal Ketone Levels

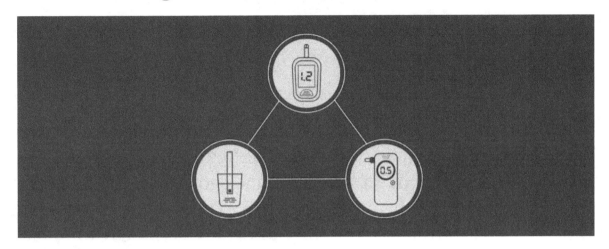

THIS PORTION IS COMPLETELY OPTIONAL. There are three different ways to test to see if you're in nutritional ketosis.

- **Blood Ketone Monitor**
- **Breath Monitor—hard to find in the US https://www.ketonix.com/**
- **Urine Strips (not as accurate, as the data is pulled from excess ketones in the urine and can be skewed by hydration levels)**

Testing can get expensive, so it's completely up to you if you choose to do it or not. Since ketones are a byproduct of fat metabolism, you can actually measure the amount of ketones that are present in your body!

If two different people consume the same exact diet of 15% carbs, 25% protein, and 60% fat, one person may be able to achieve nutritional ketosis, while the other may need to adjust the breakdown a little bit.

The only way to know for sure is to test. Be sure to carefully follow the directions that come with whichever device you decide to use.

Nutritional ketosis is achieved when you've reached between (.5-3.0 mmol/L).

Now, you should know that achieving ketosis isn't an instant thing. It can take a little while.

If you test below .5mmol/L, then you're not yet in nutritional ketosis, and you need to change up your macro breakdown.

You'll likely need to add a bit more healthy fat and consume fewer carbs and/or less protein. In fact, for some people, too much protein in the diet can knock them out of ketosis. Therefore, it's important to make sure you're not consuming too many carbs OR too much protein.

If you're reading higher than 3.0, you simply need to add a little more protein and/or carbs into your diet.

Keep this in mind: More ketones is not better! Having more than 5-6mmol/L present in your body is indicative of "starvational ketosis." This is when your body will start breaking down muscle for energy.

With this 30-day plan, I've provided you with a very moderate approach, so you shouldn't have to worry about getting too high.

When to test:

You'll find your ketones are typically highest in the morning. That's because you just fasted while you were sleeping.

You can test at various times per day—just be consistent.

You'll absolutely see phenomenal results if you stick to the plan, regardless of if you test or not.

It's just a fun and nerdy way to track exactly what is going on in your body.

Have Fun & St i c k to the Plan!

In order to get the best benefit from this transformational book, remember: you have to stick to it!

We're always here to help if you need anything. Enjoy the journey!

CHAPTER THREE

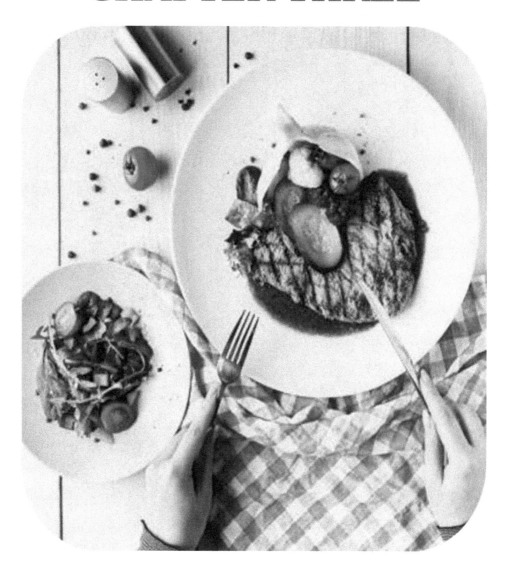

30-Day Keto Diet Weight Loss Meal Plan

The purpose of this plan is to show you what types of keto foods you can eat, ways you can prepare your foods, what a typical keto meal looks like, and recipes.

How to use this plan:

- Each day will be between 1,500–1,700 calories (designed for weight loss).

- Make sure you know your daily macros (how much fat, protein, carbs, and calories you need to achieve your goal).

- Each recipe has anywhere between 2–10 servings, so be sure to prepare according to your macros and personal needs. For example, if you only cook for yourself, you might want to make one serving at a time, or make as many servings as you want and keep the leftovers for the next few days.

- Be flexible. We don't know your personal goal, your budget, your cooking skills, what your favorite foods are, or what foods you don't like to eat, so we cannot personalize the meal plan just for you. This plan is just to give you ideas of what to cook for breakfasts, lunches, and dinners. So please feel free to adjust and personalize it to make it work for you.

- Feel free to replace any of the recipes or ingredients with your personal choices and adjust the ingredient amounts to fit your macros and situation.

WEEK 1

THIS WEEK'S MEAL PLAN

	Breakfast	Lunch	Dinner
DAY 1	Chorizo Breakfast Bake	Sesame Pork Lettuce Wraps	Avocado Lime Salmon
DAY 2	Low-Carb Breakfast Egg Muffins Filled with Sausage Gravy	Spiced Pumpkin Soup	Easy Creamy Shredded Chicken with Spinach and Bacon
DAY 3	Baked Eggs in Avocado	Easy Beef Curry	Rosemary Roasted Chicken and Veggies
DAY 5	Egg Strata with Blueberries and Cinnamon	Lettuce Rolls with Ground Beef	Homemade Sage Sausage Patties
DAY 6	Sweet Blueberry Coconut Porridge with 1 Slice Thick-Cut Bacon	Stuffed Jalapeno Peppers with Ground Beef	Sauteed Sausage with Green Beans
DAY 7	Low-Carb Breakfast Quiche	Bacon Wrapped Asparagus	Lamb Chops with Rosemary and Garlic

RECIPES FOR WEEK 1

<u>Chorizo breakfast bake</u>

Nutritional Facts Per Serving	
Calories	212
Fat	11 g
Net Carb	9 g
Total Carbs:	11 g
Fiber:	2 g
Protein	9 g

Prep Time: *10 minutes/* ***Cook Time:*** *50 minutes/* ***Servings:*** *4*

Ingredients

- 2 tablespoon olive oil
- 1 red bell pepper
- 1 yellow bell pepper
- 200 grams (7 ounces) chorizo sausage
- 6 large eggs
- 2 large red onion (cut into wedges)
- 2 cloves garlic (minced)
- ½ cup coconut milk
- Salt and pepper

Instructions

Preheat the oven to 425 degrees Fahrenheit (220 degrees Celsius).
Cut the bell peppers in half, remove the seeds and stem and place the halves on a baking tray. Drizzle with 1 tbsp olive oil and put in the oven to roast for 20 minutes. After 10 minutes of baking, place the red onion wedges on the tray, drizzle with a splash of olive oil and return to the oven to cook for another 10 minutes. The peppers are done when they are soft and have a slightly charred skin. When the peppers are done, place them on a cutting board and place a bowl overtop to trap the steam.
Leave them to rest for 5 minutes (this will make it easier to peel off the skin).
In a cast iron skillet heat 1 tbsp olive oil on medium high heat. Stir in the minced garlic and cook for 20 seconds until fragrant and then add in the chopped chorizo and cook for 5 minutes until the chorizo is cooked through and then remove from the heat.
While the chorizo is cooking peel the skin off of the roasted bell peppers. Cut the peeled peppers into thin strips.
In a bowl whisk together the eggs, coconut milk, paprika, cayenne, salt and pepper.

Add the sliced peppers and red onion to the cast iron skillet and pour the egg mixture overtop. Transfer to the oven to bake for 20-25 minutes until the egg has set and the top of the frittata is firm to the touch. Serve sprinkled with chopped parsley.

Sesame Pork Lettuce Wraps

Nutritional Facts Per Serving	
Calories	500
Fat	29 g
Net Carb	7.5 g
Total Carbs:	10.5 g
Fiber:	3 g
Protein	49 g

Prep Time: 10 minutes/ *Cook Time:* 5 minutes/ *Servings:* 2

Ingredients
- 1 tablespoon olive oil
- ¼ cup diced yellow onion
- ¼ cup diced green pepper
- 2 tablespoons diced celery
- 6 ounces ground pork
- ¼ teaspoon onion powder
- ¼ teaspoon garlic powder
- 2 tablespoons soy sauce
- 1 teaspoon sesame oil
- 4 leaves butter lettuce, separated
- 1 tablespoon toasted sesame seeds

Instructions

1. Heat the oil in a skillet over medium heat.
2. Add the onions, peppers, and celery and sauté for 5 minutes until tender.
3. Stir in the pork and cook until just browned.
4. Add the onion powder and garlic powder, then stir in the soy sauce and sesame oil.
5. Season with salt and pepper to taste, then remove from heat.
6. Place the lettuce leaves on a plate and spoon the pork mixture evenly into them.

7. Sprinkle with sesame seeds to serve.

Avocado Lime Salmon

Nutritional Facts Per Serving	
Calories	570
Fat	44 g
Net Carb	4 g
Total Carbs:	12 g
Fiber:	8 g
Protein	36 g

Prep Time: 15 minutes/ *Cook Time:* 15 minutes/ *Servings:* 2

Ingredients

- 100 grams chopped cauliflower
- 1 large avocado
- 1 tablespoon fresh lime juice
- 2 tablespoons diced red onion
- 2 tablespoons olive oil
- 2 (6-ounce) boneless salmon fillets
- Salt and pepper

Instructions

1. Place the cauliflower in a food processor and pulse into rice-like grains.
2. Grease a skillet with cooking spray and heat over medium heat.
3. Add the cauliflower rice and cook, covered, for 8 minutes until tender. Set aside.
4. Combine the avocado, lime juice, and red onion in a food processor and blend smooth.
5. Heat the oil in a large skillet over medium-high heat.
6. Season the salmon with salt and pepper, then add to the skillet skin-side down.
7. Cook for 4 to 5 minutes until seared, then flip and cook for another 4 to 5 minutes.

8. Serve the salmon over a bed of cauliflower rice topped with the avocado cream.

Low-Carb

Breakfast Egg Muffins Filled with

Sausage Gravy

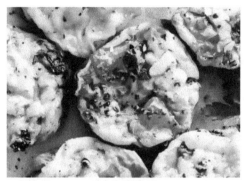

Nutritional Facts Per Serving	
Calories	607
Fat	46 g
Net Carb	3 g
Total Carbs:	6 g
Fiber:	3 g
Protein	42 g

Prep Time: 15 minutes/ *Cook Time:* 35 minutes/ *Servings:* 6

Ingredients

For the muffins:
- 12 large eggs
- Sea salt
- Black pepper
- 1 pound thin shaved deli ham
- 4 ounces shredded mozzarella cheese
- 4 ounces grated parmesan cheese
- Low-carb sausage gravy

For the gravy:
- 1/2 ground pork sausage
- 8 ounces softened cream cheese

- 3/4 cups beef broth
- Sea salt
- Black pepper

Instructions

1. Prepare the eggs and gravy.
2. Whisk eggs together with salt and pepper to taste.
3. Cook the sausage over medium heat until thoroughly cooked through.
4. Add in the cream cheese and the broth and stirring constantly, cook until the mixture comes to a soft simmer and thickens.
5. Then reduce the heat to medium-low, still stirring constantly and simmer for 2 more minutes.
6. Season to taste with salt and pepper.
7. Set mixture aside.
8. Preheat oven to 325°F.

Assemble the muffins:

- Place two pieces of ham in the bottom of each muffin cup, careful to overlap and try and cover the whole surface.
- Evenly divide sausage gravy between each muffin.
- Pour eggs into each muffin, dividing the mixture evenly.
- Top each muffin with equal parts of the two types of cheeses.
- Bake for approximately 30-40 minutes or until muffin is firm and cheese is melted.

Spiced Pumpkin Soup

Nutritional Facts Per Serving	
Calories	250
Fat	20 g
Net Carb	6 g
Total Carbs:	8 g
Fiber:	2 g
Protein	10 g

Prep Time: 15 minutes/ *Cook Time:* 40 minutes/ *Servings:* 3

Ingredients

- 2 tablespoons unsalted butr
- 1 small yellow onion, chopped
- 2 cloves minced garlic
- 1 teaspoon minced ginger
- ½ teaspoon ground cinnamon
- ¼ teaspoon ground nutmeg
- Salt and pepper, to taste
- ½ cup pumpkin puree
- 1 cup chicken broth
- 3 slices thick-cut bacon
- ¼ cup heavy cream

Instructions

1. Melt the butter in a large saucepan over medium heat.
2. Add the onions, garlic, and ginger and cook for 3 to 4 minutes until the onions are translucent.
3. Stir in the spices and cook for 1 minute until fragrant. Season with salt and pepper.
4. Add the pumpkin puree and chicken broth, then bring to a boil.
5. Reduce heat and simmer for 20 minutes, then remove from heat.

6. Puree the soup using an immersion blender, then return to heat and simmer for 20 minutes.
7. Cook the bacon in a skillet until crisp, then remove to paper towels to drain.
8. Add the bacon fat to the soup along with the heavy cream. Crumble the bacon over top to serve.

Easy Creamy Shredded Chicken with Spinach and Bacon

Nutritional Facts Per Serving	
Calories	*383*
Fat	*23.2 g*
Net Carb	*0.9 g*
Total Carbs:	*1.2 g*
Fiber:	*0.3 g*
Protein	*40.3 g*

Prep Time: *10 minutes/* ***Cook Time:*** *20 minutes/* ***Servings:*** *2*

Ingredients

- 1 chicken breast, boiled
- 1 slice bacon, chopped
- 2 tbsp butter
- 1/2 cup spinach, chopped
- 1 tbsp onion in slices
- 2 tbsp cream cheese
- 1 tsp Italian seasoning
- 1 tsp salt
- 1/2 tsp black pepper

Instructions

1. First, let the chicken boil in hot water. Afterwards, shred it with a fork or with your hands. Set aside.
2. Pan fry the chopped bacon in melted butter. When the bacon starts producing fats, gently drop the shredded chicken in and cook for 2-3 minutes.
3. Toss in the spinach and onion into the pan. Leave to soften the vegetables.
4. Mix in the cream cheese and stir continuously to blend the ingredients. Add more flavor with the Italian seasoning, pepper, and salt.

5. Transfer to a serving plate and enjoy your meal.

Baked Eggs in Avocado

Nutritional Facts Per Serving	
Calories	610
Fat	54 g
Net Carb	4.5 g
Total Carbs:	18 g
Fiber:	13.5 g
Protein	20 g

Prep Time: 5 minutes/ **Cook Time:** 15 minutes/
Servings: 2

Ingredients
- 1 medium avocado
- 2 tablespoons lime juice
- 2 large eggs
- Salt and pepper
- 2 tablespoons shredded cheddar cheese

Instructions

1. Preheat the oven to 450°F and cut the avocado in half.
2. Scoop out some of the flesh from the middle of each avocado half.
3. Place the avocado halves upright in a baking dish and brush with lime juice.
4. Crack an egg into each and season with salt and pepper.
5. Bake for 10 minutes, then sprinkle with cheese.
6. Let the eggs bake for another 2 to 3 minutes until the cheese is melted. Serve hot.

Easy Beef Curry

Nutritional Facts Per Serving	
Calories	550
Fat	34 g
Net Carb	9 g
Total Carbs:	14 g
Fiber:	5 g
Protein	50 g

Prep Time: 20 minutes/ *Cook Time:* 40 minutes/ *Servings:* 3

Ingredients

- 1 medium yellow onion, chopped
- 1 tablespoon minced garlic
- 1 tablespoon grated ginger
- 1 ¼ cups canned coconut milk
- 1 pound beef chuck, chopped
- 2 tablespoons curry powder
- 1 teaspoon salt
- ½ cup fresh chopped cilantro

Instructions

1. Combine the onion, garlic, and ginger in a food processor and blend into a paste.
2. Transfer the paste to a saucepan and cook for 3 minutes on medium heat.
3. Stir in the coconut milk, then simmer gently for 10 minutes.
4. Add the chopped beef along with the curry powder and salt.
5. Stir well then simmer, covered, for 20 minutes.
6. Remove the lid and simmer for another 20 minutes until the beef is cooked through.

Adjust seasoning to taste and garnish with fresh chopped cilantro.

Rosemary Roasted Chicken and Veggies

Nutritional Facts Per Serving	
Calories	540
Fat	40.5 g
Net Carb	8.5 g
Total Carbs:	12 g
Fiber:	3.5 g
Protein	33 g

*Prep Time: 15 minutes/ **Cook Time:** 35 minutes/ **Servings:** 2*

Ingredients

- 4 deboned chicken thighs
- Salt and pepper
- 1 small zucchini, sliced
- 2 small carrots, peeled and sliced
- 1 small parsnip, peeled and sliced
- 2 cloves garlic, sliced
- 3 tablespoons olive oil
- 1 tablespoon balsamic vinegar
- 2 teaspoons fresh chopped rosemary

Instructions

1. Preheat the oven to 350°F and lightly grease a small rimmed baking sheet with cooking spray.
2. Place the chicken thighs on the baking sheet and season with salt and pepper.
3. Arrange the veggies around the chicken then sprinkle with sliced garlic.
4. Whisk together the remaining ingredients then drizzle over the chicken and veggies.
5. Bake for 30 minutes then broil for 3 to 5 minutes until the skins are crisp.

Lemon Poppy Ricotta Pancakes

Nutritional Facts Per Serving	
Calories	370
Fat	26 g
Net Carb	5.5 g
Total Carbs:	6.5 g
Fiber:	1 g
Protein	29.5g

Prep Time: *10 minutes/* **Cook Time:** *20 minutes/* **Servings:** *2*

Ingredients

- 1 large lemon, juiced and zested
- 6 ounces whole milk ricotta
- 3 large eggs
- 10 to 12 drops liquid stevia
- ¼ cup almond flour
- 1 scoop egg white protein powder
- 1 tablespoon poppy seeds
- ¾ teaspoons baking powder
- ¼ cup powdered erythritol
- 1 tablespoon heavy cream

Instructions

1. Combine the ricotta, eggs, and liquid stevia in a food processor with half the lemon juice and the lemon zest—blend well, then pour into a bowl.
2. Whisk in the almond flour, protein powder, poppy seeds, baking powder, and a pinch of salt.
3. Heat a large nonstick pan over medium heat.
4. Spoon the batter into the pan, using about ¼ cup per pancake.
5. Cook the pancakes until bubbles form on the surface of the batter, then flip them.

6. Let the pancakes cook until the bottom is browned, then remove to a plate.
7. Repeat with the remaining batter.
8. Whisk together the heavy cream, powdered erythritol, and reserved lemon juice and zest.
9. Serve the pancakes hot, drizzled with the lemon glaze.

Keto Bunless Bacon Cheeseburger with Mushrooms

Nutritional Facts Per Serving	
Calories	627
Fat	50.7 g
Net Carb	2.2 g
Total Carbs:	3 g
Fiber:	0.8 g
Protein	39.6g

Prep Time: *5 minutes/* **Cook Time:** *15 minutes/*
Servings: *4*

Ingredients

- 1 lb ground beef
- 4 slices bacon
- 1 small egg
- 1 tbsp almond flour
- 1 tsp cumin
- 1/2 cup sliced mushrooms
- 1 tsp garlic powder
- 1 tsp onion powder
- 8 cheddar cheese thin slices
- Salt
- 1 tsp black pepper

Instructions

1. Season the ground beef with all of the condiments. Crack the egg into the beef and throw in the almond flour as well. Knead until well combined. Mold into 4 meatballs.
2. Create the hollow shape of the meatballs with a soda can. Using your hands, shape the beef to form a cup before removing the can.

3. Fill the molded beef with mushroom. Wrap a slice of bacon around the sides of the cup.
4. Lay a slice of cheese on the surface of the hamburger to cover the mushroom. Leave in the 300°F oven for 10 minutes. Remove once the meat is cooked.
5. Lay another slice of cheese on top and rebake for an additional 5 minutes, enough to melt the cheese.
6. Serve and enjoy!

Stuffed Chicken Breasts

Nutritional Facts Per Serving	
Calories	417
Fat	17.9 g
Net Carb	2.6 g
Total Carbs:	3.6 g
Fiber:	1 g
Protein	58.7g

Prep Time: 10 minutes/ *Cook Time:* 30 minutes/ *Servings:* 3

Ingredients

- 1.5 lb chicken breast, approx. 3 pcs
- 1 cup chopped spinach fresh
- 1/2 cup cherry tomatoes
- 1 garlic clove
- 6 tbsp shredded cheese
- 2 tbsp olive oil
- 1/2 cup Rao's homemade tomato basil sauce (optional)

Instructions

1. Prepare all ingredients.
2. Add one tbsp of olive oil in a skillet, add spinach, quartet cherry tomatoes, and chopped garlic. Cook it until spinach is soft.
3. Make pockets in chicken breasts. Salt, pepper, you can add Mediterranean dry herbs (basil, oregano). I had three chicken breasts so I first stuffed each with one tbsp of cheese and then cooked greens. Close cuts with wooden toothpicks.
4. Brown chicken in the skillet on both sides (don't cook it) then transfer into a deep tray with the remaining tbsp of olive oil.
5. Distribute sauce evenly on top of the chicken. Cover with foil.
6. Preheat oven to 375°F. Cook till it's done.

7. As a final step sprinkle remaining cheese on top of the chicken, send it back to oven for a few min for cheese to melt.
8. Enjoy.

Egg Strata with Blueberries and Cinnamon

	Nutritional Facts Per Serving
Calories	188
Fat	15 g
Net Carb	1 g
Total Carbs:	4 g
Fiber:	3 g
Protein	8 g

Prep Time: *5 minutes*/ **Cook Time:** *20 minutes*/ **Servings:** *4*

Ingredients

- 6 large eggs
- 2 tbsp softened butter
- 1 tsp vanilla
- 1/2 cup blueberries (or 1/4 cup, depending upon taste)
- 1/2 tsp cinnamon (you could probably double this if you like cinnamon)
- 1 tbsp coconut oil

Instructions

1. Preheat oven to 375°F.
2. In an 8" - 9" cast iron skillet (or any oven-proof skillet), heat coconut oil over medium heat.
3. In a medium bowl beat eggs, butter, cinnamon, and vanilla together with a hand mixer until combined and fluffy (about 1-2 minutes).
4. Pour egg mixture into heated pan and allow bottom to cook slightly (about 2 minutes). Gently drop blueberries into egg mixture and place pan in oven. Cook for 15-20 or until cooked through and browned on top (but not burned).
5. Remove from oven and allow to cool slightly.

Lettuce Rolls with Ground Beef

Nutritional Facts Per Serving	
Calories	127
Fat	8.5 g
Net Carb	1.4 g
Total Carbs:	2.1 g
Fiber:	0.7 g
Protein	10.6 g

Prep Time: 10 minutes/ *Cook Time:* 15 minutes/ *Servings:* 4

Ingredients

- 4 lettuce leaves
- ½ lb ground beef
- 1 tbsp olive oil
- 2 tbsp chopped onion
- 1 small tomato, chopped
- ½ tsp paprika
- 1 small avocado, chopped
- 2 tbsp sour cream
- ½ tsp salt
- ½ tsp black pepper

Instructions

1. In a hot frying pan with a tbsp of olive oil, sauté the onion and tomato. Gently plop the beef into the sautéed onion and tomato. Season with pepper, salt, paprika, and any other spice of your choice. Sear for 7-10 minutes over medium-high heat.
2. Lay the lettuce leaf on a flat board. Scoop out some of the cooked beef and place this on one side of the leaf. Top with avocado and sour cream. Roll the leaf firmly. Repeat until all of the ingredients are used up.
3. Transfer to a plate and enjoy!

Homemade Sage Sausage Patties

Nutritional Facts Per Serving	
Calories	162
Fat	11 g
Carbohydrates:	1 g
Protein	13 g

Cook Time: *15 minutes/* **Servings:** *8*

Ingredients

- 1 pound ground pork
- 3/4 cup shredded cheddar cheese
- 1/4 cup buttermilk
- 1 tablespoon finely chopped onion
- 2 teaspoons rubbed sage
- 3/4 teaspoon salt
- 3/4 teaspoon pepper
- 1/8 teaspoon garlic powder
- 1/8 teaspoon dried oregano

Instructions

1. In a bowl, combine all ingredients, mixing lightly but thoroughly. Shape into eight 1/2-inch-thick patties. Refrigerate 1 hour.
2. In a large cast-iron or other heavy skillet, cook patties over medium heat until a thermometer reads 160° 6-8 minutes on each side.

Sweet Blueberry Coconut Porridge

Nutritional Facts Per Serving	
Calories	390
Fat	22 g
Net Carb	15 g
Total Carbs:	37 g
Fiber:	22 g
Protein	10 g

Prep Time: 5 minutes/ *Cook Time:* 15 minutes/ *Servings:* 2

Ingredients

- 1 cup unsweetened almond milk
- ¼ cup canned coconut milk
- ¼ cup coconut flour
- ¼ cup ground flaxseed
- 1 teaspoon ground cinnamon
- ¼ teaspoon ground nutmeg
- Pinch salt
- 60 grams fresh blueberries
- ¼ cup shaved coconut

Instructions

1. Warm the almond milk and coconut milk in a saucepan over low heat.
2. Whisk in the coconut flour, flaxseed, cinnamon, nutmeg, and salt.
3. Turn up the heat and cook until the mixture bubbles.
4. Stir in the sweetener and vanilla extract, then cook until thickened to the desired level.
5. Spoon into two bowls and top with blueberries and shaved coconut.

Stuffed Jalapeno Peppers with Ground Beef

Nutritional Facts Per Serving	
Calories	127
Fat	8.5 g
Net Carb	1.4 g
Total Carbs:	2.1 g
Fiber:	0.7 g
Protein	10.6 g

Prep Time: 15 minutes/ *Cook Time:* 30 minutes/ *Servings:* 6

Ingredients

- 6 large jalapeños
- 1 tbsp olive oil
- ½ lb ground beef
- 2 tbsp chopped onion
- 1 small tomato, chopped
- 2 oz grated mozzarella cheese
- ½ tsp salt
- ½ tsp black pepper

Instructions

1. While preparing the dish, let the oven preheat at 350°F.
2. Heat the olive oil in a frying pan. Sauté the beef in the pan together with the onion and chopped tomato. Add salt and pepper to taste. Leave to cook for approximately 15 minutes.
3. Slice the jalapeños into two pieces. Empty the insides of the slices by discarding the seeds and the veins.
4. Stuff about a tablespoonful of the cooked beef in the empty jalapeño halves. Sprinkle mozzarella cheese on the surface. Arrange the filled peppers on a baking sheet and cook in the oven for 15 minutes. Wait till the cheese browns.
5. Serve on a plate and enjoy!

Sauteed Sausage with Green Beans

Nutritional Facts Per Serving	
Calories	369
Fat	32.6 g
Net Carb	3.6 g
Total Carbs:	4.5 g
Fiber:	0.9 g
Protein	15 g

*Prep Time: 15 minutes/ **Cook Time:** 15 minutes/ **Servings:** 3*

Ingredients

- 300 g pork sausage
- 1/2 cup green beans
- 1/2 onion, sliced
- 1/2 tbsp olive oil
- 2 tbsp sour cream
- Salt and pepper, to taste

Instructions

1. Chop off both tips of the green beans then slice into two. Put aside.
2. Chop the sausage links into bite-sized chunks as well. Reserve in a bowl. For easy chopping, refrigerate the sausage for around 15 minutes before cutting.
3. Preheat a skillet then pour the oil into heat. Sear the sausage chunks for 5 minutes.
4. Once brown, toss in the onion and chopped green beans. Sauté for 4-5 minutes more.
5. Gently pour in the cream. Season with pepper and salt. Fold the mix with a spatula to incorporate all the ingredients together. Leave for an additional 3 minutes before turning off the heat.
6. Serve in a dish and enjoy warm.

Low-Carb Breakfast Quiche

Nutritional Facts Per Serving	
Calories	551
Fat	46 g
Net Carb	3 g
Total Carbs:	6 g
Fiber:	3 g
Protein	26 g

Prep Time: 15 minutes/ **Cook Time:** 55 minutes/ **Servings:** 4

Ingredients

- 1 lb ground Italian sausage
- 1.5 cups shredded cheddar cheese
- 8 large eggs
- 1 tbsp ranch seasoning
- 1 cup sour cream

Instructions

1. Preheat oven to 350°F.
2. In an oven-safe skillet, brown ground sausage and drain the grease.
3. In a large bowl, whisk together egg, sour cream, and ranch seasoning. You may want to use a hand mixer.
4. Mix in cheddar cheese.
5. Pour egg mixture into pan and stir until everything is fully blended.
6. Cover with foil and bake for 30 minutes.
7. Remove foil and bake for another 25 minutes or until golden brown.

Bacon Wrapped Asparagus

Nutritional Facts Per Serving	
Calories	565
Fat	54.6 g
Net Carb	2.8 g
Total Carbs:	4.8 g
Fiber:	2 g
Protein	15 g

Prep Time: *5 minutes/* ***Cook Time:*** *20 minutes/* ***Servings:*** *2*

Ingredients

- 12 spear fresh asparagus, medium-sized
- 2 tbsp olive oil
- 6 slices bacon
- Salt and black pepper, to taste

Instructions

1. Set the oven to 350°F to preheat.
2. After rinsing the asparagus with water, chop off the tough parts of the stem.
3. Drizzle olive oil on the asparagus spears. Salt and pepper to enhance the flavor. Wrap half a strip of bacon around each asparagus. Repeat until all the ingredients are used up.
4. Arrange the wrapped asparagus on a baking sheet in a way that they don't overlap. Leave in the oven for 20 minutes. Wait till the vegetable is tender.
5. Transfer to a plate. Best served warm.

Lamb Chops with Rosemary and Garlic

Nutritional Facts Per Serving	
Calories	685
Fat	52 g
Net Carb	3 g
Total Carbs:	6 g
Fiber:	3 g
Protein	50.5 g

Prep Time: 35 minutes/ *Cook Time:* 15 minutes/ *Servings:* 2

Ingredients

- 1 tablespoon coconut oil, melted
- 1 teaspoon fresh chopped rosemary
- 1 clove garlic, minced
- 2 bone-in lamb chops (about 6 ounces meat)
- 1 tablespoon butter
- Salt and pepper
- ¼ pound fresh asparagus, trimmed
- 1 tablespoon olive oil

Instructions

1. Combine the coconut oil, rosemary, and garlic in a shallow dish.
2. Add the lamb chops then turn to coat – let marinate in the fridge overnight.
3. Let the lamb rest at room temperature for 30 minutes.
4. Heat the butter in a large skillet over medium-high heat.
5. Add the lamb chops and cook for 6 minutes, then season with salt and pepper.
6. Turn the chops and cook for another 6 minutes or until cooked to the desired level.
7. Let the lamb chops rest for 5 minutes before serving.
8. Meanwhile, toss the asparagus with olive oil, salt, and pepper then spread on a baking sheet.

9. Broil for 6 to 8 minutes until charred, shaking occasionally. Serve hot with the lamb chops.

WEEK 2

THIS WEEK'S MEAL PLAN

	Breakfast	Lunch	Dinner
DAY 8	Fat-Busting Vanilla Protein Smoothie	Easy Cheeseburger Salad	Chicken Zoodle Alfredo
DAY 9	Savory Ham and Cheese Waffles with 2 Slices Thick-Cut Bacon	Pan-Fried Pepperoni Pizzas	Cabbage and Sausage Skillet
DAY 10	Mozzarella Veggie-Loaded Quiche with 1 Slice Thick-Cut Bacon	Keto Fried Chicken Tenders with Almond Flour	Gyro Salad with Avo-Tzatziki
DAY 11	Pepper Jack Sausage Egg Muffins with 3 Slices Thick-Cut Bacon	Bacon Burger Bites	Chicken Alfredo with Broccoli
DAY 12	Broccoli Cheesy Bread	Keto Salmon Sushi Rolls	Buffalo Chicken Wings
DAY 13	Avocado Smoothie with Coconut Milk	Pan Fried Spinach Stuffed Chicken	Low-Carb Nachos
DAY 14	Coconut Flour Pancakes	Crustless Pizza in a Bowl	Keto Chicken Cordon Bleu

RECIPES FOR WEEK 2

Fat-Busting Vanilla Protein Smoothie

Nutritional Facts Per Serving	
Calories	540
Fat	46 g
Net Carb	7.5 g
Total Carbs:	8 g
Fiber:	0.5 g
Protein	25 g

Prep Time: *5 minutes/* ***Cook Time:*** *none/* ***Servings:*** *2*

Ingredients

- 1 scoop (20g) vanilla egg white protein powder
- ½ cup heavy cream
- ¼ cup vanilla almond milk
- 4 ice cubes
- 1 tablespoon coconut oil
- 1 tablespoon powdered erythritol
- ½ teaspoon vanilla extract
- ¼ cup whipped cream

Instructions

1. Combine all of the ingredients, except the whipped cream, in a blender.
2. Blend on high speed for 30 to 60 seconds until smooth.
3. Pour into a glass and top with whipped cream.

Easy Cheeseburger Salad

Nutritional Facts Per Serving	
Calories	395
Fat	27.5 g
Net Carb	8 g
Total Carbs:	9 g
Fiber:	1 g
Protein	27.5 g

Prep Time: 10 minutes/ **Cook Time:** 10/ *Servings:* 2

Ingredients

- 7 ounces ground beef
- Salt and pepper
- 3 tablespoons mayonnaise
- 1 tablespoon diced pickles
- 1 teaspoon mustard
- ½ teaspoon ketchup
- Pinch smoked paprika
- 3 ounces chopped romaine lettuce
- 1/3 cup diced tomatoes
- ¼ cup shredded cheddar cheese

Instructions

1. Brown the ground beef over high heat then season with salt and pepper to taste.
2. Drain the fat from the beef and remove from heat.
3. Combine the mayonnaise, pickles, mustard, ketchup, and paprika in a blender.
4. Blend the mixture until smooth and well combined.
5. Combine the lettuce, tomatoes, and cheddar cheese in a mixing bowl.
6. Toss in the ground beef and the dressing until evenly coated.

Chicken Zoodle Alfredo

Nutritional Facts Per Serving	
Calories	595
Fat	40 g
Net Carb	3 g
Total Carbs:	4 g
Fiber:	1 g
Protein	55 g

Prep Time: 10 minutes/ **Cook Time:** *25/* **Servings:** *2*

Ingredients

- 2 (6-ounce) chicken breasts
- 1 tablespoon olive oil
- Salt and pepper
- 2 tablespoons butter
- ¼ cup heavy cream
- ¼ cup grated Parmesan cheese
- 200 grams zucchini

Instructions

1. Heat the oil in a large skillet over medium-high heat.
2. Season the chicken with salt and pepper to taste then add to the skillet.
3. Cook for 6 to 7 minutes on each side until cooked through then slice into strips.
4. Reheat the skillet over medium-low heat and add the butter.
5. Stir in the heavy cream and Parmesan cheese then cook until thickened.
6. Spiralize the zucchini then toss it into the sauce mixture with the chicken.
7. Cook until the zucchini is tender, about 2 minutes, then serve hot.

Savory Ham and Cheese Waffles

Nutritional Facts Per Serving	
Calories	575
Fat	46.5 g
Net Carb	5 g
Total Carbs:	5 g
Fiber:	0 g
Protein	35 g

Prep Time: *15 minutes/* ***Cook Time:*** *25/* ***Servings:*** *2*

Ingredients

- 4 large eggs, divided
- 2 scoops (40 g) egg white protein powder
- 1 teaspoon baking powder
- 1/3 cup melted butter
- ½ teaspoon salt
- 1 ounce diced ham
- ¼ cup shredded cheddar cheese

Instructions

1. Separate two of the eggs and set the other two aside.
2. Beat 2 of the egg yolks with the protein powder, baking powder, butter, and salt in a mixing bowl.
3. Fold in the chopped ham and grated cheddar cheese.
4. Whisk the egg whites in a separate bowl with a pinch of salt until stiff peaks form.
5. Fold the beaten egg whites into the egg yolk mixture in two batches.
6. Grease a preheated waffle maker then spoon ¼ cup of the batter into it and close it.
7. Cook until the waffle is golden brown, about 3 to 4 minutes, then remove.
8. Reheat the waffle iron and repeat with the remaining batter.

9. Meanwhile, heat the oil in a skillet and fry the eggs with salt and pepper.
10. Serve the waffles hot, topped with a fried egg.

Pan-Fried Pepperoni Pizzas

Nutritional Facts Per Serving	
Calories	545
Fat	42 g
Net Carb	4.5 g
Total Carbs:	12 g
Fiber:	7.5 g
Protein	32 g

Prep Time: *10 minutes/* ***Cook Time:*** *25/* ***Servings:*** *3*

Ingredients

- 6 large eggs
- 6 tablespoons grated Parmesan cheese
- 3 tablespoons psyllium husk powder
- 1 ½ teaspoons Italian seasoning
- 3 tablespoons olive oil
- 9 tablespoons low-carb tomato sauce, divided
- 4 ½ ounces shredded mozzarella, divided
- 1 ½ ounces diced pepperoni, divided
- 3 tablespoons fresh chopped basil

Instructions

1. Combine the eggs, Parmesan, and psyllium husk powder with the Italian seasoning and a pinch of salt in a blender.
2. Blend until smooth and well combined, about 30 seconds, then rest for 5 minutes.
3. Heat 1 tablespoon of oil in a skillet over medium-high heat.
4. Spoon 1/3 of the batter into the skillet and spread in a circle then cook until browned underneath.
5. Flip the pizza crust and cook until browned on the other side.
6. Remove the crust to a foil-lined baking sheet and repeat with the remaining batter.
7. Spoon 3 tablespoons of low-carb tomato sauce over each crust.

8. Top with diced pepperoni and shredded cheese then broil until the cheese is browned.
9. Sprinkle with fresh basil then slice the pizza to serve.

Cabbage and Sausage Skillet

Nutritional Facts Per Serving	
Calories	350
Fat	24.5 g
Net Carb	10 g
Total Carbs:	12 g
Fiber:	2 g
Protein	22 g

Prep Time: 10 minutes/ *Cook Time:* 20/ *Servings:* 4

Ingredients

- 6 large Italian sausage links
- ½ head green cabbage, sliced
- 2 tablespoons butter
- ¼ cup sour cream
- ¼ cup mayonnaise
- Salt and pepper

Instructions

1. Cook the sausage in a skillet over medium-high heat until evenly browned then slice them.
2. Reheat the skillet over medium-high heat then add the butter.
3. Toss in the cabbage and cook until wilted, about 3 to 4 minutes.
4. Stir the sliced sausage into the cabbage then stir in the sour cream and mayonnaise.
5. Season with salt and pepper then simmer for 10 minutes.

Mozzarella Veggie-Loaded Quiche

Nutritional Facts Per Serving	
Calories	590
Fat	40 g
Net Carb	17 g
Total Carbs:	24.5 g
Fiber:	7.5 g
Protein	38 g

*Prep Time: 10 minutes/ **Cook Time:** 25/ **Servings:** 3*

Ingredients

- 6 tablespoons almond flour
- 1 tablespoon grated Parmesan cheese
- 2 large eggs, divided
- 2 slices thick-cut bacon
- ¼ cup frozen spinach, thawed and drained well
- ¼ cup diced zucchini
- ¼ cup shredded mozzarella cheese
- 4 cherry tomatoes, halved
- 1 tablespoon heavy cream
- 1 teaspoon chopped chives

Instructions

1. Stir together the almond flour and grated Parmesan with one egg and a pinch of salt until it forms a soft dough.
2. Press the dough into the bottom of a small quiche pan as evenly as possible.
3. Score the bottom and sides of the dough then bake for 7 minutes at 325°F and let cool.
4. Cook the bacon in a skillet until browned then crumble and spread in the quiche pan.
5. Sprinkle in the spinach, zucchini, cheese, and tomatoes.

6. Whisk together the remaining egg with the heavy cream, chives, salt and pepper then pour into the quiche. Bake for 22 to 25 minutes until the egg is set then serve hot.

Keto Fried Chicken Tenders with Almond Flour

Nutritional Facts Per Serving	
Calories	236
Fat	10.7 g
Net Carb	2.1 g
Total Carbs:	2.9 g
Fiber:	0.8 g
Protein	30.1 g

*Prep Time: 10 minutes/ **Cook Time:** 15/ **Servings:** 4*

Ingredients

- 500 g chicken breast
- 1 cup almond flour
- 1/4 cup sour cream
- 1 tbsp lemon juice
- 1 large egg
- 2 cloves garlic
- 1/2 tsp chili powder (optional)
- 1 tsp salt
- 1/2 tsp pepper
- Coconut oil for frying

Instructions

1. Slice your chicken breast to produce lengthwise ribbons.
2. Smash the spices and garlic clove in a mortar. Coat the chicken with the crushed spices and garlic. Crack the egg in the chicken bowl. Mix together with the sour cream and lemon juice. Fold gently to drench the chicken in the seasonings.
3. Cover the chicken with the lid and chill in the fridge for about an hour, flipping the pieces occasionally to marinate thoroughly. After an hour, remove the liquid to make sure the meat is not too wet and soggy.

4. Pour the almond flour in a container with a lid. Transfer the seasoned chicken into the container. Replace the lid and shake well to coat the chicken with enough flour.
5. Set a deep fryer to 375°F and pour in the oil.
6. Once the oil becomes hot enough, deep fry the chicken strips for 10-15 minutes. Serve immediately once the strips become golden.

Gyro Salad with Avo-Tzatziki

Nutritional Facts Per Serving	
Calories	495
Fat	29 g
Net Carb	7.5 g
Total Carbs:	13.5 g
Fiber:	6 g
Protein	45 g

Prep Time: *10 minutes/* **Cook Time:** *25/* **Servings:** *3*

Ingredients

- 1 tablespoon olive oil
- 1 pound ground lamb meat
- ½ medium yellow onion, diced
- ¼ cup chicken broth
- 4 teaspoons lemon juice, divided
- ½ teaspoon dried oregano
- ½ teaspoon dried thyme
- ½ English cucumber
- 1 medium ripe avocado
- 2 teaspoons fresh chopped mint
- 1 teaspoon fresh chopped dill
- 6 cups chopped romaine lettuce

Instructions

1. Heat the oil in a large skillet over medium-high heat and add the lamb.
2. Cook for 3 minutes, stirring often, then stir in the onion.
3. Keep cooking until the lamb is cooked through and the onion softened then stir in the chicken broth, 2 teaspoons lemon juice, oregano, and thyme.
4. Season with salt and pepper to taste then simmer for 5 minutes.

5. Grate the cucumber then spread evenly on a clean towel and wring out the moisture.
6. Place the grated cucumber in a food processor and add the avocado, 2 teaspoons lemon juice, mint, and dill with a pinch of salt. Blend the mixture until smooth.
7. Serve the gyro meat over chopped lettuce with a spoonful of avo-tzatziki.

Pepper Jack Sausage Egg Muffins

Nutritional Facts Per Serving	
Calories	455
Fat	37 g
Net Carb	3 g
Total Carbs:	3.5 g
Fiber:	0.5 g
Protein	26 g

Prep Time: *10 minutes/* **Cook Time:** *30/* **Servings:** *3*

Ingredients

- 10 ounces ground breakfast sausage
- ½ cup diced yellow onion
- ¼ teaspoon garlic powder
- Salt and pepper
- 3 large eggs, whisked
- 2 tablespoons heavy cream
- ½ cup shredded pepper jack cheese

Instructions

1. Preheat the oven to 350°F and grease three ramekins with cooking spray.
2. Stir together the ground sausage, diced onion, garlic powder, salt, and pepper in a mixing bowl.
3. Divide the sausage mixture evenly in the ramekins, pressing it into the bottom and sides, leaving the middle open.
4. Whisk together the eggs and heavy cream with salt and pepper.
5. Divide the egg mixture among the sausage cups and top with shredded cheese.
6. Bake for 25 to 30 minutes until the eggs are set and the cheese browned.

Bacon Burger Bites

Nutritional Facts Per Serving	
Calories	173
Fat	14.1 g
Net Carb	0.6g
Total Carbs:	0.7 g
Fiber:	0.1 g
Protein	10.4 g

Prep Time: *10 minutes/* **Cook Time:** *15/* **Servings:** *16*

Ingredients

- 1 lb ground beef
- 8 slices bacon, halved
- 1 large egg, beaten
- 1/2 cup almond flour
- 1/2 tsp garlic powder
- 6 slices mozzarella cheese
- Pickled Jalapeños (optional)
- Salt and pepper, to taste

Instructions

1. Season the meat with garlic powder, salt, and pepper. Crack the egg on the meat and mix well with the almond flour. Knead with your hands or with a spoon to flavor it entirely and create a consistent mixture.
2. Mold into 16 mini meatballs.
3. Prepare 8 strips of bacon and divide into two, making 16 bacon slices. Wrap one slice around one ball.
4. Crispy fry the bacon in two tablespoons of oil using a nonstick frying pan. Remember to cook all sides of the balls.
5. Transfer to a dish once the meatballs turn golden on every side and the bacon is crispy to your liking.

6. Slice the jalapeno into slivers and the cheese into small squares.

7. Top the hot meatballs with a piece of cheese and a slice of jalapeno. Push a toothpick through the ball to hold the tower together. Let the cheese melt on top of the meatball.

8. Enjoy warm with any dip of your choice!

Chicken Alfredo with Broccoli

Nutritional Facts Per Serving	
Calories	311
Fat	19.5 g
Net Carb	2.5g
Total Carbs:	3.3 g
Fiber:	0.8 g
Protein	31.1 g

Prep Time: *10 minutes/* **Cook Time:** *15/* **Servings:** *4*

Ingredients

- 1 lb boneless chicken breast, cut in slices
- 1/2 cup spinach, cut in slices
- 1 cup broccoli florets
- 4 slices bacon (fried and cut into crisp bacon bits)
- 1 tbsp butter
- 1/2 cup heavy cream
- 1 garlic clove minced
- 2 tbsp onion, chopped
- 1/2 tsp salt
- 1/2 tsp pepper

Instructions

1. Give the broccoli the right tenderness and color by placing them in a bowl and pouring some boiling water in. Leave for 10 minutes.
2. On a hot frying pan, sauté the chicken in melted butter with the garlic and onion for 5 minutes.
3. Gently plop the spinach and broccoli into the pan. Add the bacon and cream as well. Season with salt and pepper to your liking. Leave for another 5 minutes.
4. Pour in a bowl and serve warm.

Broccoli Cheesy Bread

Nutritional Facts Per Serving	
Calories	*258*
Fat	*18.7 g*
Net Carb	*4.1g*
Total Carbs:	*6.2 g*
Fiber:	*2.1 g*
Protein	*17.4 g*

Prep Time: 10 minutes/ *Cook Time:* 15/ *Servings:* 4

Ingredients

- 3 cups broccoli
- 1 large egg
- ¼ cup Parmesan cheese, freshly grated
- 1 ½ cup cheddar cheese, shredded
- 2 tsp almond flour
- ½ tsp garlic powder
- Kosher salt
- Black pepper

Instructions

1. Wash and dry your fresh broccoli bunch. Discard all of the leaves before chopping into chunks. Make sure to chop enough chunks for 3 cups.
2. Transfer the chopped broccoli pieces into a food processor. Continue pulsing until you get rice-size bits.
3. Set the microwave to "cooking." Leave the broccoli rice in the microwave for a minute and a half.
4. Crack the egg in a bowl. Add the garlic, cheddar cheese, and almond flour together with the riced broccoli. Beat with a spoon until combined. Season with a dash of pepper and salt.

5. Pat the mixture into a baking tray covered with waxed paper. Cover all sides of the tray evenly.

6. Sprinkle a generous amount of Parmesan cheese on top. Put in the oven for 10 minutes. The oven should be set at 300°F.

7. Take the tray out of the oven. Top with half a cup of cheddar cheese. Rebake for 5 more minutes to melt the cheese.

8. Once ready, remove from the heat. Allow cooling for around 5 minutes then remove the paper.

9. Cut into rectangular shapes and enjoy!

Keto Salmon Sushi Rolls

Nutritional Facts Per Serving	
Calories	310
Fat	24 g
Net Carb	5.1g
Total Carbs:	9.3 g
Fiber:	4.2 g
Protein	16.4 g

Prep Time: 20 minutes/ Cook Time: 20/ Servings: 4

Ingredients

Sushi Fillings:
- 2 eggs
- 120 g fresh salmon (or smoked salmon)
- 100 g avocado (1 small)
- 100 g cucumber (1 small)

Sushi Rice:
- 3 cup cauliflower rice (shredded cauliflower)
- 150 g cream cheese, softened
- 2 tbsp rice vinegar
- 1/2 tsp salt, to taste
- 1/2 tsp So Nourished Erythritol (optional)

Other ingredients:
- 2 sheets Nori
- 2 tbsp white sesame seeds
- 1 tsp black sesame seeds (for decoration, optional)
- Sushi dip (optional)
- 1 tbsp ginger, grated
- 1 tbsp lemon juice
- 2 tbsp coconut aminos

Instructions
Making vinegared sushi rice

1. Wash and cut the cauliflower into small pieces to prepare the cauliflower rice. You can use a knife or a food processor (better choice) to process until obtaining the rice-like pieces.
2. Place the riced cauliflower in a closed container and cook it in the microwave for three minutes. Allow them to cool down. You can also steam or cook the cauliflower in a frying pan.
3. In a mixing bowl, add rice vinegar, sweetener, and salt. Add cauliflower rice and cream cheese in. Stir everything well with a wooden spoon until you obtain a homogeneous dough.

Prepare sushi fillings and assemble

4. Peel off the avocado and cucumber skins. Slice into slivers. Slice the salmon into thin slivers too. Scramble egg with a pinch of salt, fry it in a pan, then cut into thin strips.
5. Prep a sushi roller with transparent plastic on both sides to avoid sticking the mixture onto the roller.
6. Place the sushi mat roller on a flat surface. Lay a rectangular nori sheet on top.
7. Split the rice mixture into 2 parts for the 2 nori sheets. Scoop out one part and spread this mixture uniformly over the nori sheet.
8. Arrange the strips of avocado, salmon, egg, and cucumber on one short edge of the sheet. Make sure that the roller can be reeled in that direction.
9. With extra care, roll the filled side up to the other edge of the sheet. Repeat the procedure with the other sheets and remaining mixture.
10. Ideally, chill in the fridge for half an hour before cutting the roll. If desired, simply slice the roll without refrigerating. Slice all sushi rolls into bite-size pieces. This should make 4 servings.

Sushi dip (optional)

11. Start making the dip by pouring the lemon juice and coconut aminos in a small pot.
12. Toss in the ginger. Let it boil until the sauce darkens and intensifies in color.
13. Transfer to a small dish and place aside the sushi.

14. Enjoy!

Buffalo Chicken Wings

Nutritional Facts Per Serving	
Calories	300
Fat	17.8 g
Net Carb	3.4 g
Total Carbs:	7.1 g
Fiber:	3.7 g
Protein	28.6 g

Prep Time: *10 minutes/* **Cook Time:** *15/* **Servings:** *4*

Ingredients

- 12 chicken wings (whole wings)
- 4 cloves garlic, peeled
- 2 tbsp coconut flour
- 50 ml hot sauce
- 1 tbsp vinegar
- 1 tbsp pepper
- 1 tbsp paprika
- ½ tbsp celery salt
- 1 pinch Stevia (optional)
- 1 lemon (optional)
- Olive oil for deep frying
- 1 tsp salt
- 1 tsp chili pepper

Instructions

1. Coat the chicken wings with lemon on all sides. Set aside for 3 minutes, then wash and dry thoroughly. For a simpler method, just wash and dry the wings without putting in the lemon.
2. Smash together the paprika, pepper, garlic, salt, hot pepper, hot sauce, and vinegar with a mortar

3. Marinate the chicken wings with the mixed spices. Chill in the fridge for an hour while flipping the wings occasionally.
4. Transfer the wings to a plate and coat with coconut flour all over to cover the entire sides.
5. Pour the oil in a deep fryer set at 375°F.
6. Brown the wings in the oil for around 10-15 minutes.
7. Remove from the heat once the wings turn brown on the sides. Serve on a platter.

Avocado Smoothie with Coconut Milk

Nutritional Facts Per Serving	
Calories	283
Fat	25.3 g
Net Carb	4.5 g
Total Carbs:	14.4 g
Fiber:	9.9 g
Protein	3.2 g

Prep Time: *10 minutes/ **Cook Time:** 5/ **Servings:** 1*

Ingredients

- 1 cup coconut milk, unsweetened
- 1 tsp ginger, fresh and grounded
- 1/2 avocado
- 5 leaves spinach
- 1 tsp lime juice (optional)
- 1 tsp Stevia (optional)
- 1 tsp chia seeds

Instructions

1. Wash your ginger and spinach thoroughly.
2. Peel the ginger and avocado. Slice them into pieces.
3. Using a blender, mix all of the ingredients (except chia seeds and stevia) for a minute to obtain a smooth and uniform mixture. Optionally, pour some water and lime juice into the blender to produce the desired thickness.
4. Include some ice cubes and the sweetener into the mix just to flavor it up. Transfer to a glass and garnish with a teaspoon of chia seeds on top. Serve immediately.

Pan Fried Spinach Stuffed Chicken

Nutritional Facts Per Serving	
Calories	291
Fat	13.1 g
Net Carb	0.9 g
Total Carbs:	1.2 g
Fiber:	0.3 g
Protein	41.7 g

Prep Time: *10 minutes/* **Cook Time:** *20/* **Servings:** *2*

Ingredients

- 1 chicken breast, boneless and skinless
- 1/2 cup chopped spinach
- 1 tbsp onion, chopped
- 1 tbsp butter
- Oil for frying
- 2 tbsp cream cheese
- 1 tbsp grated mozzarella cheese
- Salt and pepper, to taste

Instructions

1. Melt your butter in a hot frying pan. Sauté the spinach and onion in the butter. Set the stove to medium-high heat and leave the vegetables to cook for about 3 minutes until soft.
2. Mix the cream cheese in the pan. Allow dissolving for around 2 minutes. Stir to combine with the onion and spinach. Set aside.
3. Slice a pocket in the chicken breast, deep enough to be filled. Rub both sides of the chicken with salt and pepper. Season all side, including the inside of the pocket.
4. Jampack the pocket with spinach filling and some shredded cheese. Close the breast and secure with a toothpick.
5. Heat the olive oil in a frying pan over medium heat. Gently place the chicken on the oil and cook for 7-10 minutes with the lid on.

Turn the chicken over and let it fry for another 7-10 minutes. Remove from the heat once golden.

6. Cut in the middle to spill the filling. Enjoy while warm.

Low-Carb Nachos

Nutritional Facts Per Serving	
Calories	507
Fat	42.1 g
Net Carb	4.9 g
Total Carbs:	10.5 g
Fiber:	5.6 g
Protein	26.1 g

Prep Time: *20 minutes/* **Cook Time:** *25/* **Servings:** *4*

Ingredients

For the chips:

- ½ cup almond flour
- 4 slices cheddar cheese (can also use grated mozzarella cheese)
- 2 tbsp butter, melted
- 2 tbsp cream cheese
- 1 small egg (optional)
- 1 tsp salt

For topping

- 1/2 lb ground beef
- 1/2 tsp dried oregano
- 1 small tomatoes, chopped
- 1 clove garlic, minced
- 1/2 tsp ground pepper
- 2 bay leaves (optional)

For guacamole

- 1 avocado medium-sized, peeled and chopped
- 1 tbsp fresh cilantro, chopped
- 1 small tomato, chopped
- 1 tbsp onion, chopped

Instructions

1. Preheat oven to 350°F.

2. Mix the almond flour, butter, oregano, cream cheese, oregano, and 1 tsp salt in a bowl. Make sure to mix until the dough looks soft so you can use a rolling pin to flatten the dough.
3. Cut small rectangles to form the crackers and place cheddar cheese on each cracker. Place them on a baking sheet and then in the oven for about 10 minutes or until they look brown. Set aside.
4. In the meantime, add oil to a preheated skillet and add the garlic clove, bay leaves, ground beef, pepper, and salt. Let it cook for 10 minutes and then add 2 chopped tomatoes. Cook for 5 more minutes and remove from heat.
5. For the guacamole, mix the avocado, 1 chopped tomato, cilantro, and onion. Add salt to taste.
6. Serve nacho crackers with meat and sour cream on top along with guacamole and enjoy!

Coconut Flour Pancakes

Nutritional Facts Per Serving	
Calories	274
Fat	23.39 g
Net Carb	4.24 g
Total Carbs:	8.04 g
Fiber:	3.8 g
Protein	8.44 g

*Prep Time: 10 minutes/ **Cook Time:** 10/ **Servings:** 2*

Ingredients

Main Ingredients:

- 2 tbsp coconut flour
- 2 eggs
- ½ tbsp So Nourished Erythritol or a dash of stevia extract
- ¼ tsp baking powder
- 2 tbsp sour cream
- 2 tbsp melted butter
- ½ tsp vanilla extract

For the topping:

- 50 g strawberries
- 1 tbsp shredded coconut
- 1 tbsp almond slices
- 1 tbsp maple syrup (optional)

Instructions

1. Put the eggs, sour cream, 1 ½ tbsp. of melted butter (you'll need the rest for frying the pancakes), vanilla extract, and mix well.
2. Add the coconut flour, baking powder, erythritol to the mixture and mix again. Let the mixture sit for about 15 minutes. If the mixture is too thick, add a little bit of water (20-30 ml) and mix again until the consistency is right.

3. In a pan on medium heat, add butter in and fry the pancakes in butter. The number of pancakes you make will depend on the size you want. We made 6 pancakes with this recipe.
4. Add the toppings and serve!

Crustless Pizza in a Bowl

Nutritional Facts Per Serving	
Calories	213
Fat	15.9 g
Net Carb	5.3 g
Total Carbs:	7 g
Fiber:	1.7 g
Protein	11.7 g

Prep Time: *5 minutes/* **Cook Time:** *10/* **Servings:** *1*

Ingredients

- 1/2 green bell pepper, cut in slices
- 1 oz turkey ham, cut in small squares
- 1 tbsp red onion, cut in slices
- 2 tbsp Rao's Pizza Sauce (or tomato paste)
- 1/2 tbsp olive oil
- 1 oz grated mozzarella cheese

Instructions

1. Preheat a frying pan then pour the oil in. Fry the ham for 3 minutes. Optionally, use any meat of your choice instead of ham. Put aside.
2. Set the bell pepper on the base of a microwave-safe bowl. Layer with the onion, ham and finally, tomato paste.
3. Top with mozzarella.
4. Microwave for 3 minutes and let the cheese melt. As an alternative, bake for 10 minutes in the oven preheated at 370°F. Remember to use an oven-safe pan for this.
5. Take out from the microwave (or oven) and enjoy!!

Keto Chicken Cordon Bleu

Nutritional Facts Per Serving	
Calories	356
Fat	19.3 g
Net Carb	1.5 g
Total Carbs:	1.7 g
Fiber:	0.2 g
Protein	42.5 g

Prep Time: *5 minutes/* **Cook Time:** *15/* **Servings:** *2*

Ingredients

- 1 pc chicken breast, boneless and skinless
- 1 lemon (optional)
- 3 slices bacon
- 1 clove garlic, minced
- 1 slice smoked ham
- 1 slice cheddar cheese
- Lettuce (optional)
- Salt and pepper, to taste

Instructions

1. Spray all the sides of the chicken breast with lemon. Set aside for 3 minutes then wash and dry the chicken thoroughly. If there are no lemons available, simply wash and towel dry.
2. Season the chicken with salt, pepper, and minced garlic. Slice the cheese and ham enough to cover the chicken.
3. Lay the ham and cheese slices on top of each chicken breast. Carefully roll the chicken, tuck the ends inside, and finally hold the pieces together with a toothpick.
4. Prepare 3 strips of bacon and wrap them around the rolled up chicken breast.
5. Set an 8-inch non-stick skillet sprayed with cooking spray over medium-high heat.

6. Sear the chicken in the pan, 5 minutes per side until there are no more pink spots on the chicken.
7. Leave in the pan for an additional 2 minutes before removing the toothpick. Lay the chicken on top of a bed of lettuce and serve.
8. If preferred, make the breadcrumb coating for the chicken. Brush the cooked chicken with beaten egg (1 egg or less) and roll it in 2-3 tbsp of almond flour to coat entirely. Crispy fry for 3 minutes until brown.

WEEK 3

THIS WEEK'S MEAL PLAN

	Breakfast	Lunch	Dinner
DAY 15	Corned Beef and Radish Hash	Mozzarella Tuna Melt	Cheesy Single-Serve Lasagna
DAY 16	Southwestern Omelet	Avocado, Egg & Salami Sandwiches	Crispy Chipotle Chicken Thighs
DAY 17	Three-Cheese Pizza Frittata with 3 Slices Thick-Cut Bacon	Stuffed Mushrooms with Bacon and Cheese	Pepperoni, Ham, and Cheddar Stromboli
DAY 18	Low-Carb Bagels with Almond Flour	Zucchini Pasta with Chicken	Low-Carb Tacos with Cheese Shells
DAY 19	Farmer Cheese Pancakes	Tahini Egg Salad with Mayonnaise	Jalapeno Popper Chicken Casseroles
DAY 20	Eggs and Asparagus Breakfast Bites	Lasagna Cabbage Rolls	Spring Salad with Steak and Sweet Dressing
DAY 21	Avocado Breakfast Muffins	Mushroom Soup with Fried Egg and 2 Slices Thick-Cut Bacon	Lasagna Stuffed Peppers

RECIPES FOR WEEK 3

Corned Beef and Radish Hash

Nutritional Facts Per Serving	
Calories	252
Fat	16 g
Carbohydrates	2 g
Protein	23 g

Cook Time: *20/* **Servings:** *4*

Ingredients

- 1 tablespoon olive oil
- 1/4 cup diced onions
- 1 cup radishes, diced to about 1/4 inch
- 1/2 teaspoon kosher salt
- 1/4 teaspoon ground black pepper
- 1/2 teaspoon dried oregano (Mexican if you have it)
- 1/4 teaspoon garlic powder
- 1 - 12 ounce can corned beef or 1 cup finely chopped corned beef, packed

Instructions

1. Heat the olive oil in a large saute pan and add the onions, radishes, salt, and pepper.
2. Saute the onions and radishes on medium heat for 5 minutes or until softened.

3. Add the oregano, garlic powder, and corned beef to the pan and stir well until combined.
4. Cook over low to medium heat, stirring occasionally for 10 minutes or until the radishes are soft and starting to brown.
5. Press the mixture into the bottom of the pan and cook on high heat for 2-3 minutes or until the bottom is crisp and brown.
6. Serve hot.

Mozzarella Tuna Melt

Nutritional Facts Per Serving	
Calories	550
Fat	36 g
Net Carb	10.5 g
Total Carbs:	11.5 g
Fiber:	1 g
Protein	45 g

Prep Time: 10 minutes/ **Cook Time:** 10/ *Servings:* 2

Ingredients

- 1 tablespoon olive oil
- ½ cup diced yellow onion
- 8 ounces canned tuna
- ¼ cup mayonnaise
- 2 large eggs, whisked
- 2 ounces shredded mozzarella cheese
- Salt and pepper
- 1 green onion, sliced thin

Instructions

1. Heat the oil in a skillet over medium heat.
2. Add the onion and cook until translucent, about 5 minutes.
3. Drain the tuna, then flake it into the skillet and stir in the remaining ingredients.
4. Season with salt and pepper and cook for 2 minutes or until the cheese melts.
5. Spoon into a bowl and top with sliced green onion to serve.

Cheesy Single-Serve Lasagna

Nutritional Facts Per Serving	
Calories	325
Fat	19 g
Net Carb	8.5 g
Total Carbs:	10 g
Fiber:	1.5 g
Protein	29 g

Prep Time: 15 minutes/ *Cook Time:* 5/ *Servings:* 4

Ingredients

- 3 tablespoons low-carb marinara sauce
- 1 small zucchini (60g), sliced very thin into rounds
- 2 tablespoons ricotta cheese
- 3 ounces shredded mozzarella
- Dried oregano

Instructions

1. Spoon 1 tablespoon marinara sauce into a microwave-safe bowl.
2. Spread one third of the zucchini slices over the sauce, then cover with a tablespoon of ricotta.
3. Repeat the layers of sauce, zucchini, and ricotta.
4. Top with the remaining zucchini and the last tablespoon of marinara.
5. Sprinkle with mozzarella then microwave for 3 to 4 minutes until the entire mixture is heated through and the cheese is melted.
6. Sprinkle with dried oregano and serve hot.

Southwestern Omelet

Nutritional Facts Per Serving	
Calories	390
Fat	31 g
Carbohydrates	7 g
Protein	22 g

Cook Time: 10/ Servings: 4

Ingredients

- 1/2 cup chopped onion
- 1 jalapeno pepper, minced
- 1 tablespoon canola oil
- 6 large eggs, lightly beaten
- 6 bacon strips, cooked and crumbled
- 1 small tomato, chopped
- 1 ripe avocado, cut into 1-inch slices
- 1 cup shredded Monterey Jack cheese, divided
- Salt and pepper, to taste

- Salsa (optional)

Instructions

1. In a large skillet, saute onion and jalapeno in oil until tender; remove with a slotted spoon and set aside. Pour eggs into the same skillet; cover and cook over low heat for 3-4 minutes.
2. Sprinkle with the onion mixture, bacon, tomato, avocado, and 1/2 cup cheese. Season with salt and pepper.
3. Fold omelet in half over filling. Cover and cook for 3-4 minutes or until eggs are set.
4. Sprinkle with remaining cheese. Serve with salsa if desired.

Avocado Egg & Salami Sandwiches

Nutritional Facts Per Serving	
Calories	490
Fat	40,5 g
Net Carb	5 g
Total Carbs:	12,5 g
Fiber:	7.5 g
Protein	22.5 g

Prep Time: 10 minutes/ Cook Time: 10/ Servings: 2

Ingredients

- 4 Easy Cloud Buns
- 1 teaspoon butter
- 4 large eggs
- 1 medium tomato, sliced into 4 slices
- 1 ounce fresh mozzarella, sliced thin
- 1 small avocado, sliced thin
- 2 ounces sliced salami
- Salt and pepper

Instructions

1. Toast the cloud buns on a baking sheet in the oven until golden brown.
2. Heat the butter in a large skillet over medium heat.
3. Crack the eggs into the skillet and season with salt and pepper.
4. Cook the eggs until done to the desired level then place one on each cloud bun.
5. Top the buns with sliced tomato, mozzarella, avocado, and salami.

Crispy Chipotle Chicken Thighs

Nutritional Facts Per Serving	
Calories	400
Fat	20 g
Net Carb	1,5 g
Total Carbs:	3 g
Fiber:	1.5 g
Protein	51 g

Prep Time: *15 minutes/* ***Cook Time:*** *15/* ***Servings:*** *3*

Ingredients

- ½ teaspoon chipotle chili powder
- ¼ teaspoon garlic powder
- ¼ teaspoon onion powder
- ¼ teaspoon ground coriander
- ¼ teaspoon smoked paprika
- 12 ounces boneless chicken thighs
- Salt and pepper
- 1 tablespoon olive oil
- 3 cups fresh baby spinach

Instructions

1. Combine the chipotle chili powder, garlic powder, onion powder, coriander, and smoked paprika in a small bowl.
2. Pound the chicken thighs out flat, then season with salt and pepper on both sides.
3. Cut the chicken thighs in half and heat the oil in a heavy skillet over medium-high heat.
4. Add the chicken thighs skin-side-down to the skillet and sprinkle with the spice mixture.
5. Cook the chicken thighs for 8 minutes then flip and cook on the other side for 3 to 5 minutes.

6. During the last 3 minutes, add the spinach to the skillet and cook until wilted. Serve the crispy chicken thighs on a bed of wilted spinach.

Three-Cheese Pizza Frittata

Nutritional Facts Per Serving	
Calories	305
Fat	24 g
Net Carb	2,5 g
Total Carbs:	3.5 g
Fiber:	1 g
Protein	21 g

Prep Time: 10 minutes/ *Cook Time:* 40/ *Servings:* 4

Ingredients

- ½ (10-ounce) bag frozen spinach, thawed
- 6 large eggs
- 2 tablespoons olive oil
- ½ teaspoon dried Italian seasoning
- Salt and pepper
- ¼ cup ricotta cheese
- ¼ cup grated Parmesan cheese
- 2 ½ ounces shredded mozzarella cheese
- 1 oz sliced pepperoni

Instructions

1. Preheat the oven to 375°F and grease a pie plate with cooking spray.
2. Defrost the frozen spinach in the microwave for 4 minutes, then squeeze out the water.
3. Whisk together the eggs, olive oil, Italian seasoning, salt, and pepper in a bowl.
4. Stir in the ricotta cheese, Parmesan cheese, and drained spinach until well combined.
5. Pour the mixture into the pie plate and top with mozzarella and pepperoni.

6. Bake for 35 to 40 minutes until the egg is set and the cheese lightly browned.

Stuffed Mushrooms with Bacon and Cheese

Nutritional Facts Per Serving	
Calories	306
Fat	24.5 g
Net Carb	5 g
Total Carbs:	6.4 g
Fiber:	1,4 g
Protein	16,3 g

Prep Time: *10 minutes/* **Cook Time:** *10/* **Servings:** *3*

Ingredients

- 12 large mushrooms, stems removed and chopped
- 3 slices bacon
- 1 egg
- 1 onion, chopped
- Olive oil for cooking spray
- 1 tsp coriander, chopped
- 1 clove garlic
- 1 tsp chilli pepper (optional)
- 3 slices cheddar cheese
- Salt and ground black pepper, to taste

Instructions

1. Let the oven preheat at 300°F while preparing the dish.
2. Wash the mushrooms thoroughly, then cut out the stem. Chop the stem into small pieces before putting aside.
3. Set an 8-inch non-stick skillet coated with cooking spray over medium-high heat. Sauté the onion and garlic in the skillet and brown the bacon as well.
4. Crack the egg in a mixing bowl. Toss in the cooked garlic, onion, and bacon. Add the grated cheese, chopped mushroom stem, and coriander into the mixing bowl. Stir the ingredients well. Adjust the flavor with some salt and pepper.

5. Scoop out a teaspoonful of the mixed ingredients and stuff it inside the mushroom caps.
6. Place in the oven and leave to bake for around 25 minutes till the surface of the caps turns golden. Serve on a platter.

Pepperoni, Ham & Cheddar Stromboli

Nutritional Facts Per Serving	
Calories	525
Fat	37 g
Net Carb	8 g
Total Carbs:	16 g
Fiber:	8 g
Protein	32 g

Prep Time: 20 minutes/ *Cook Time:* 20/ *Servings:* 3

Ingredients

- 1 ¼ cups shredded mozzarella cheese
- ¼ cup almond flour
- 3 tablespoons coconut flour
- 1 teaspoon dried Italian seasoning
- Salt and pepper
- 1 large egg, whisked
- 6 ounces sliced deli ham
- 2 ounces sliced pepperoni
- 4 ounces sliced cheddar cheese
- 1 tablespoon melted butter
- 6 cups fresh salad greens

Instructions

1. Preheat the oven to 400°F and line a baking sheet with parchment.
2. Melt the mozzarella cheese in a microwave-safe bowl until it can be stirred smooth.
3. In a separate bowl, stir together the almond flour, coconut flour, and dried Italian seasoning.
4. Pour the melted cheese into the flour mixture and mix it with some salt and pepper.
5. Add the egg and work it into a dough then put it onto a piece of parchment.

6. Lay a piece of parchment on top and roll the dough out into an oval.
7. Use a knife to cut diagonal slits along the edges, leaving the middle 4 inches untouched.
8. Layer the ham and cheese slices in the middle of the dough then fold the strips over the top.
9. Brush the top with butter, then bake for 15 to 20 minutes until the dough is browned. Slice the Stromboli and serve with a small salad.

Low-Carb Bagels with Almond Flour

	Nutritional Facts Per Serving
Calories	396
Fat	54 g
Net Carb	7 g
Protein	17 g

Prep Time: *10 minutes/* **Cook Time:** *20/* **Servings:** *6*

Ingredients
Dough:

- 3 cups shredded mozzarella

- 4 tbsp cream cheese
- 2 eggs
- 2 tsp xanthan gum
- 1.5 cups almond flour

Toppings (to taste):

- Poppy seeds
- Sesame seeds
- Garlic powder
- Onion Powder

Instructions

1. While preparing the dough, preheat the oven to 400°F.
2. Crack the eggs in a bowl and beat it well with the xanthan gum and almond flour.
3. Melt the cream cheese and mozzarella together in a pot set over low heat.
4. Pour the melted cheese in the almond flour mixture.

5. Knead the dough thoroughly. After a while, use a mixer to combine the ingredients since the xanthan powder, flour, and eggs can become difficult to mix.
6. Mold the dough to form log shapes, then arrange them on the donut pan. Dust with your favorite toppings.
7. Brown them in the oven for 18 minutes.
8. Serve on a plate.

Zucchini Pasta with Chicken

Nutritional Facts Per Serving	
Calories	409
Fat	26,5 g
Net Carb	7.8 g
Total Carbs:	10.9 g
Fiber:	3.1 g
Protein	33,6 g

*Prep Time: 15 minutes/ **Cook Time: 10/ Servings: 2***

Ingredients

- 2 oz chicken breast
- 1 large zucchini
- 1 tomato
- 1/2 small onion
- 2 cloves garlic, minced
- 2 tbsp olive oil
- 2 slices cheddar cheese
- 1 tbsp chopped cilantro
- Salt, to taste
- 1 tsp black pepper

Instructions

1. Slice the chicken breast to make small strips. Place in a bowl with the minced garlic, pepper, and salt. Let it marinate.
2. Pan fry the chicken in olive oil on a large skillet placed over medium heat. Leave for 5-7 minutes until tender and cooked enough.
3. Drop the tomato and onion into the pan. Cook for 3 more minutes. Let it become saucy and juicy before removing from the heat.
4. Chop off the tips of the zucchini. Grate the vegetable by pushing along on the grater starting from the top. This will create long, slim ribbons similar to a pasta noodle. Flip the zucchini and

continue grating until the zucchini is all used up. Throw away the seeds. Alternatively, create zucchini spirals with a spiralizer.

5. Boil the zoodles in a pot of hot water for about a minute. Strain then set aside. As an option, instead of boiling the noodles, stir-fry in olive oil for around 2 minutes.

6. Fry the cheese in a preheated skillet to make the cheese crisps. Allow it to melt and brown on the edges.

7. Transfer the zoodles in a plate. Top with the cheese crisps and chicken. Garnish with chopped cilantro and slices of tomato.

8. Serve and enjoy.

Low-Carb Tacos with Cheese Shells

Nutritional Facts Per Serving	
Calories	394
Fat	27,3 g
Net Carb	1.9 g
Total Carbs:	3.1 g
Fiber:	1.2 g
Protein	33 g

Prep Time: 10 minutes/ *Cook Time:* 10/ *Servings:* 4

Ingredients

For topping:
- 1/2 lb ground beef
- 1 clove garlic
- 1 slice bacon (crispy, cooked)
- 1/3 cup avocado, chopped
- 1/3 cup tomato, cut in brunoise
- 1/4 cup onion, cut in brunoise
- Salt and pepper, to taste
- 1 tsp taco seasoning (keto-friendly)
- 1 tbsp jalapenos slices (optional)
- Mayonnaise for topping (optional)

For cheese shells:
- 4 slices cheddar cheese

Instructions

1. Heat the oil in a pan and add the onion and garlic, sprinkle with taco seasoning, salt, and pepper. Add the meat then cook gently for 5 minutes, or until browned, stirring occasionally.
2. Spray 8-inch (20 cm) non-stick skillet with cooking spray and heat over medium-high heat and add bacon until it's cooked and remove from heat. Chop it into small crispy bacon bits for topping.

3. Cut onion, tomato, and avocado into small pieces for topping.
4. Spray 8-inch (20 cm) non-stick skillet with cooking spray and heat over medium-high heat and add the cheese, when the cheese is completely cooked at the bottom, you can now flip it carefully and fry the opposite side until they're brown. You can also bake the cheese in the oven as well instead of frying it.
5. Next, remove cheese from heat and put on a plate. If you want to make the taco shell shape, bend the cheese carefully while it's still warm, soft and moldable. As the cheese cools down, the shell will become hardened.
6. Place beef, avocado, tomato, purple onion, and bacon pieces and sprinkle with chili pepper and salt. You can add mayonnaise and sour cream as well.

Farmer Cheese Pancakes

Nutritional Facts Per Serving	
Calories	198
Fat	12,1 g
Net Carb	0.9 g
Total Carbs:	2.2 g
Fiber:	1.3 g
Protein	18.4 g

Prep Time: *5 minutes/* **Cook Time:** *15/* **Servings:** *4*

Ingredients

- 1 lb Farmer Cheese
- 1 cup coconut flour
- 2 eggs
- Pinch of salt, to taste (optional)
- 1 tsp Stevia, to taste (optional)

Instructions

1. Mix farmer cheese, coconut flour, salt, and 2 eggs. Mixture should be like paste texture.
2. Form pancakes into round shape. Dust it just a bit with coconut flour.
3. Fry till both sides are golden brown.

Note: Can be served with blueberries or any topping of your choice.

Tahini Egg Salad with Mayonnaise

Nutritional Facts Per Serving	
Calories	314
Fat	28,12 g
Net Carb	1.53 g
Total Carbs:	2.73 g
Fiber:	1.2 g
Protein	12.76 g

Prep Time: *5 minutes/* *Cook Time:* *5/* *Servings:* *2*

Ingredients

- 4 medium eggs, hard boiled
- 1 tbsp tahini sesame seeds paste
- 3 tbsp mayonnaise
- 1 tbsp lemon juice, freshly squeezed
- 1 tsp dijon mustard
- ¼ tsp paprika (optional)
- Salt, to taste
- Ground black pepper, to taste

Instructions

1. Prepare a bowl to combine the tahini, mayonnaise, mustard, lemon juice, and black pepper in. Stir well until incorporated.
2. Slice the boiled eggs into pieces and gently plop them into the bowl.
3. Fold the egg thoroughly into the mixture. Sprinkle ¼ tsp of paprika on the surface if preferred.
4. Serve and enjoy.

Jalapeno Popper Chicken Casserole

Nutritional Facts Per Serving	
Calories	498
Fat	35,7 g
Net Carb	3.2g
Total Carbs:	3.7 g
Fiber:	0.5 g
Protein	39.6 g

Prep Time: 10 minutes/ *Cook Time:* 40/ *Servings:* 6

Ingredients

- 1 lb chicken breast, cooked
- 4 slices bacon
- 1 tbsp butter
- 4 jalapenos (up to your liking)
- 3 cloves garlic
- 1/2 cup onion, diced
- 1/2 cup chicken broth
- 1 cup cream cheese
- 2 cup cheddar cheese, divided
- 2 tablespoons fresh coriander
- Salt and pepper, to taste

Instructions

1. Preheat the oven to 200 °C (400°F).
2. Cut the precooked chicken breast into small bite-sized pieces and set aside. (Note: If you don't have precooked chicken breast ready, simply prepare this by seasoning raw chicken breast with salt, pepper, lemon juice, and olive oil then bake at 400°F for 25-30 minutes until cooked).
3. Chop bacon slices, garlic, and onion with a sharp knife into small pieces. Sauté them with butter in a large frying pan or a wok over medium heat. Fry until the onion and the bacon are translucent. This could take about 10 minutes.

4. Add jalapeno slices, coriander, salt, and pepper. Stir well for 2 minutes.
5. Add cream cheese, half of the cheddar cheese, and chicken broth. Bring to boil, then simmer. Stir gently for about 10 minutes until you get a thick and creamy mixture.
6. Making the casserole: Place chicken pieces at the bottom of a casserole or a baking dish. Pour the cream cheese mixture on top of the chicken and finally add the remaining cheddar cheese. Bake in the oven for about 15-20 minutes or until the cheese is all melted.
7. Top with a few pieces of jalapenos, crispy bacon bits, and coriander. Serve warm with a low-carb salad or leafy greens.

Eggs and Asparagus Breakfast Bites

Nutritional Facts Per Serving	
Calories	426
Fat	35,64 g
Net Carb	3.64g
Total Carbs:	5.94 g
Fiber:	2.3 g
Protein	20.73 g

Prep Time: *5 minutes/* ***Cook Time:*** *20/* ***Servings:*** *2*

Ingredients

- 4 medium eggs
- 100 g asparagus, fresh or canned
- 1 tbsp butter, melted
- ¼ tsp baking powder
- 1 tbsp coconut flour
- 80 g cream cheese
- 40 g shredded cheddar cheese
- Salt, to taste

Instructions

1. For fresh asparagus, chop them into about 2-cm long pieces. Pan fry for around 5 minutes in melted butter. For canned asparagus, simply chop them into pieces. Reserve.
2. Combine the rest of the ingredients in a bowl. Stir well to mix together. Put aside for 10 minutes.
3. Brush a decent amount of oil in the baking molds. Place some pieces of asparagus in the molds then add the combined mixture you reserved earlier. Avoid filling up to the brim.
4. Place in the oven set at 350°F for 20 minutes, checking occasionally if the bites are cooked thoroughly.
5. Serve on a plate and enjoy.

Lasagna Cabbage Rolls

Nutritional Facts Per Serving	
Calories	190
Fat	12,4 g
Net Carb	5.8g
Total Carbs:	8.5 g
Fiber:	2.7 g
Protein	12.5 g

Prep Time: *10 minutes/* **Cook Time:** *30/* **Servings:** *4*

Ingredients

- ½ lb ground beef, preferably sirloin ground beef
- 5 small tomatoes
- ½ tbsp dried basil
- ¼ cup cilantro, chopped
- 1 in onion slices
- 1 garlic clove, minced
- ¼ cup mushrooms, in slices
- 1 tbsp olive oil
- 3 cups water
- 8 cabbage leaves
- 1 tbsp salt
- ¼ tbsp ground pepper

Instructions

1. Boil 2 cups of water in a cooking pot. Lay the cabbage in a heat-safe bowl and gently pour the boiling water on the cabbage. Set aside for 10 minutes.
2. Heat a tbsp of oil in a frying pan. Sauté the minced garlic and half of the onion slices till they start to look soft. Add the ground beef into the pan. Flavor the mix with pepper and half a tbsp of salt. Leave to cook for 15 minutes then reserve for later.

3. Pour a cup of water in another pot while cooking the beef. Throw in the chopped cilantro, tomatoes, and the remaining onion slices. Boil the ingredients up to 15 minutes. Afterwards, transfer to a blender. Whisk together with the dried basil and another half tbsp of salt. Blend to obtain a smooth, uniform mixture for the sauce.

4. Lay a cabbage leaf on a plate. Spread spoonfuls of meat on the leaf, then add the mushrooms as well. Fold all the sides securely so the fillings will not spill. Do the same with the rest of the ingredients.

5. Set your available oven to 350°F to preheat. Lay the cabbage bites on a baking sheet and bake for 10 minutes, enough to warm them up.

6. Spread some sauce on top of the bites and serve.

Spring Salad with Steak & Sweet Dressing

Nutritional Facts Per Serving	
Calories	575
Fat	43,5 g
Net Carb	2.5g
Total Carbs:	6.5 g
Fiber:	4 g
Protein	41 g

Prep Time: 10 minutes/ *Cook Time:* 25/ *Servings:* 2

Ingredients

- 2 slices thick-cut bacon
- 2 tablespoons white wine vinegar
- 2 tablespoons olive oil
- 2 tablespoons fresh raspberries
- Liquid stevia, to taste
- 4 cups fresh spring greens
- 1 ounce toasted pine nuts
- 1 tablespoon butter
- 7 ounces beef flank steak

Instructions

1. Cook the bacon in a skillet over medium-high heat until very crisp, then chop fine. Combine the white wine vinegar, olive oil, raspberries, and liquid stevia in a blender.
2. Blend the ingredients until smooth and well combined.
3. Combine the spring greens, roasted pine nuts, and crumbled bacon in a large bowl.
4. Toss with the dressing, then divide between two plates.
5. Melt the butter in a heavy skillet over medium-high heat then add the steak.
6. Season with salt and pepper then sear on one side, about 3 to 4 minutes.

7. Flip the steak and cook to the desired level, then rest for 5 minutes.
8. S l ice the steak and divide it between the salads.

Avocado Breakfast Muffins

Nutritional Facts Per Serving	
Calories	248
Fat	19 g
Net Carb	0.9g
Total Carbs:	2.3 g
Fiber:	1,4 g
Protein	17.3 g

Prep Time: *10 minutes/* **Cook Time:** *20/* **Servings:** *20*

Ingredients

- 20 beef patties (small size, about 50 g each)
- 10 eggs, medium-sized
- 1/2 cup heavy cream
- 2 avocados, cubed
- 10 oz cheddar cheese, cubed
- Black pepper, to taste

Instructions

1. Preheat oven to 350°F.
2. Take a large muffin tin and put one sausage patty in each cup, shaping with a shot glass to line the entire inside.
3. Evenly divide the avocado and cheese in the cups.
4. Beat eggs and heavy cream together in a bowl, then pour into each cup until cheese and avocado are covered. Top with black pepper to taste.
5. Bake for 20 minutes at 350°; if desired, broil for an additional 1-2 minutes until top is browned. Enjoy!

Mushroom Soup with Fried Egg

Nutritional Facts Per Serving	
Calories	385
Fat	31 g
Net Carb	7 g
Total Carbs:	10 g
Fiber:	3 g
Protein	20 g

Prep Time: 5 minutes/ **Cook Time:** 15/ *Servings:* 2

Ingredients

- 1 teaspoon olive oil
- 4 white mushrooms, sliced thin
- 100 grams cauliflower, riced
- 1 cup vegetable broth
- 3 tablespoons heavy cream
- 2 tablespoons shredded cheese
- 1 teaspoon butter
- 1 large egg

Instructions

1. Heat the oil in a small saucepan over medium heat.
2. Add the mushrooms and cook until they are tender, about 6 minutes.
3. Stir in the riced cauliflower, vegetable broth, and heavy cream.
4. Season with salt and pepper then stir in the cheese.
5. Simmer the soup until it thickens to the desired level then remove from heat.
6. Fry the egg in the butter until cooked to the desired level then serve over the soup.

Lasagna Stuffed Peppers

Nutritional Facts Per Serving	
Calories	454
Fat	28.5 g
Net Carb	8 g
Total Carbs:	11 g
Fiber:	3 g
Protein	38.4 g

Prep Time: 10 minutes/ *Cook Time:* 30/ *Servings:* 4

Ingredients

- 4 bell peppers, large
- 1 lb ground beef
- 4 cloves garlic
- 2/3 cup marinara sauce
- 1 cup ricotta cheese
- 1.5 cup mozzarella cheese
- 1 tsp Italian seasoning
- Salt and pepper, to taste

Instructions

1. Preheat oven to 375°F.
2. Brown beef and garlic cloves. Stir in tomato sauce and ricotta cheese. Season to taste with Italian seasoning, salt, pepper, crushed red pepper flakes, etc.
3. Cut and blanch peppers for 5 minutes in boiling water. Stuff with beef and ricotta mixture. Top with mozzarella and bake for 30-35 minutes.
4. Enjoy!

WEEK 4

THIS WEEK'S MEAL PLAN

	Breakfast	Lunch	Dinner
DAY 22	Baked Avocado Eggs	Pesto Chicken with Mozzarella	Baked Shrimp with Asparagus
DAY 23	Stuffed Portobello Mushrooms	Cheddar Biscuits	Keto Eggplant Lasagna
DAY 24	Bacon and Mushroom Omelette	Zucchini Taco Bites	Grilled Beef Steak
DAY 25	Keto Deviled Eggs	Broccoli and Shrimp Sautéed in Butter	Fat Head Pizza
DAY 26	Keto Bread with Almond and Coconut Flour	Easy Cloud Buns	Chicken Breast with Eggplant, Zucchini and Spinach
DAY 27	Scrambled Eggs with Mushrooms and Cottage Cheese	Low Carb Tortillas with Ground Beef	Grilled Stuffed Zucchini with Bacon
DAY 28	Vegetable Tart	Coconut Flour Pizza Bites	Zucchini Noodles with Meatballs

RECIPES FOR WEEK 4

Baked Avocado Eggs

Nutritional Facts Per Serving	
Calories	423
Fat	41.3 g
Net Carb	2.4 g
Total Carbs:	9.5 g
Fiber:	7.1 g
Protein	7.7 g

*Prep Time: 10 minutes/ **Cook Time:** 15/ **Servings:** 2*

Ingredients

- 1 avocado, sliced in half
- 3 tbsp butter, melted
- 2 eggs whole
- 1 tsp dried oregano
- ½ tsp Himalayan Salt

Instructions

1. While preheating the oven to 400°F, prepare a small baking dish covered with parchment paper. Put aside.
2. Cut the avocado into two and remove the seed. Coat the surface with melted butter. Lay the avocado halves on the baking dish and gently crack an egg on each top. Flavor with some oregano and salt.
3. Let it cook in the oven for 15 minutes or so, depending on how cooked you like your eggs.
4. Serve in a plate and enjoy.

Pesto Chicken with Mozzarella

Nutritional Facts Per Serving	
Calories	421
Fat	25.99 g
Net Carb	1.3 g
Total Carbs:	1.7 g
Fiber:	0.4 g
Protein	43.43 g

Prep Time: 5 minutes/ *Cook Time:* 20/ *Servings:* 3

Ingredients
- 450 g chicken breast
- 5 tbsp pesto sauce
- 60 g mozzarella whole milk, shredded

Instructions

1. Set the oven to 392°F to preheat while making the dish.
2. Chop the washed chicken into small portions. You should cut about 2-3 pieces from each chicken breast.
3. Put 2 tbsp of pesto in a pan sprayed with cooking oil.
4. Throw in the chicken pieces and add the remaining pesto on top of the meat.
5. Enclose the pan with aluminum foil and allow cooking for 15 minutes or up till the meat is slightly cooked through.
6. Sprinkle the grated mozzarella on the chicken. Remove the foil completely and cook for additional 4-5 minutes.
7. Serve in a plate and enjoy.

Baked Shrimp with Asparagus

Nutritional Facts Per Serving	
Calories	278
Fat	15.88 g
Net Carb	2.62 g
Total Carbs:	3.62 g
Fiber:	1 g
Protein	25.9 g

*Prep Time: 5 minutes/ **Cook Time:** 14/ **Servings:** 2*

Ingredients

- 250 g shrimp, cleaned
- 100 g asparagus fresh or canned
- 2-3 slices lemon (optional)
- 1 tsp lemon juice
- 2 tbsp butter, melted
- 3 tbsp Parmesan, grated
- Salt, to taste

Instructions

1. Let the oven preheat at 392°F.
2. Arrange the asparagus and shrimp in an adapted container. Lay some slices of lemon on top if desired. Leave in the oven for 10 minutes to bake.
3. Check if the shrimp has turned pink and opaque. If so, drizzle the melted butter on top of the shrimp and sprinkle the grated Parmesan on the asparagus. Rebake for 5 more minutes. Wait till the cheese has melted.
4. Transfer the shrimp and asparagus on a plate and enjoy.

Stuffed Portobello Mushrooms

Nutritional Facts Per Serving	
Calories	232
Fat	16.4 g
Net Carb	6.8 g
Total Carbs:	8.5 g
Fiber:	1.7 g
Protein	15.4 g

Prep Time: 5 minutes/ *Cook Time:* 20/ *Servings:* 2

Ingredients

- 8 oz Portobello mushrooms
- 4 oz mozzarella cheese
- 4 oz cherry tomatoes
- ½ tsp balsamic vinegar for sprinkling
- 1/2 tbsp olive oil for brushing

Instructions

1. Coat the entire mushrooms with olive oil. Brush all sides and edges.
2. Dice the mozzarella and place them in the mushroom.
3. Half the cherry tomatoes and season them with the wine vinegar, salt, and pepper. Mix it with chopped basil if available. Place the seasoned tomatoes on top of the cheese.
4. Bake in the oven preheated at 375°F for 20 minutes.
5. Best served with mixed greens.

Cheddar Biscuits

Nutritional Facts Per Serving	
Calories	284
Fat	25.4 g
Net Carb	1.1 g
Total Carbs:	1.5 g
Fiber:	0.4 g
Protein	12.9 g

Prep Time: 5 minutes/ *Cook Time:* 15/ *Servings:* 4

Ingredients

- 1 cup cheddar cheese, shredded
- 1/4 cup butter melted and slightly cooled
- 4 eggs
- 1/3 cup coconut flour
- 1/4 teaspoon baking powder
- 1/4 teaspoon garlic powder
- 1 teaspoon dried parsley (optional)
- 1/4 teaspoon Old Bay Seasoning (optional)
- 1/4 teaspoon salt

Instructions

1. Set the oven to 400°F to preheat.
2. Crack the eggs in a bowl. Add the garlic powder, melted butter, dried parsley, and seasoning powder if you have some. Salt to taste.
3. Combine the cheese into the mixture together with the baking powder and coconut flour. Fold until you obtain a lump-free mixture.
4. Grease a cookie sheet before adding the batter into it. Place ice cream-size scoops into the sheet.
5. Lightly brown the biscuits in the oven for 15 minutes.
6. Serve with any meal or eat them alone.

If you like to keep them for later, allow them to cool completely before storing in a jar to preserve the crispness.

Keto Eggplant Lasagna

Nutritional Facts Per Serving	
Calories	**498**
Fat	**33.7 g**
Net Carb	**6.4 g**
Total Carbs:	**12.6 g**
Fiber:	**6.2 g**
Protein	**36.3 g**

Prep Time: *30 minutes/* ***Cook Time:*** *25/* ***Servings:*** *6*

Ingredients

- 1 lb ground beef
- 2 eggplants, medium-sized
- 6 slices bacon, chopped
- 2 cloves garlic, minced
- 1 onion small, minced
- 1 cup marinara sauce
- 1/3 cup Parmesan cheese
- 8 slices cheddar cheese
- 1 tsp oregano
- 1-2 tsp salt, to taste
- 1/2 tsp black pepper

Instructions

1. Preheat oven to 375°F.
2. In a saucepan over medium-high heat, add a little bit of oil in to fry the bacon. Once the bacon turns golden and crispy, remove and chop into small bite-sizes and set aside.
3. Use the same saucepan with the bacon fat, toss in garlic and onion. Continue frying until they soften.
4. Gently throw the ground beef into the pan. Season with salt, pepper, and oregano. Stir with a spoon and allow it cook till golden.

5. Add the marinara sauce in and bring to a boil then simmer until the volume decreases by about a third.

6. Meanwhile, peel off the eggplant skin. Cut the eggplant lengthwise into ¼ inch thin slices. Grill on a non-stick preheated pan and make sure both sides are cooked. This is an optional step just to give the lasagna a firmer consistency and intensify the amazing smell of grilled eggplant.

7. Prepare a baking dish to layer your lasagna. Place a layer of eggplant as the base, then spread the cooked beef and bacon on top of the eggplant then top with cheese. Repeat the layers until you fill the whole dish.

8. Spread more Parmesan cheese on the final layer. Bake in the oven for about 20-30 minutes until the cheese melts and the surface produces nice golden bubbles.

Remove from oven and allow cooling for about 5 minutes. Slice out a piece and enjoy with some green veggies.

Bacon and Mushroom Omelette

Nutritional Facts Per Serving	
Calories	313
Fat	23.8 g
Net Carb	1.4 g
Total Carbs:	1.6 g
Fiber:	0.2 g
Protein	22.8 g

Prep Time: 5 minutes/ *Cook Time:* 5/ *Servings:* 2

Ingredients

- 3 medium mushrooms, raw
- 2 slices bacon
- 3 eggs
- 2 tbsp onion, chopped
- 2 slices cheddar cheese
- Lettuce or watercress, to taste (optional)
- Pinch salt
- Pinch pepper

Instructions

1. Brunoise cut the onion. Slice the mushrooms and bacon into small chunks as well.
2. Heat an 8-inch non-stick skillet coated with cooking spray over medium-high heat. Cook the onion and bacon in the pan. Once the bacon is toasted enough, toss in the mushrooms and remove from the heat.
3. Beat the eggs in a mixing bowl. Flavor with sea salt and black pepper then add the cooked bacon, mushroom, and onion.
4. Gently pour the egg mixture into the pan. Once the omelette starts to firm up, ease around the edges with a spatula. Lay the slices of cheddar cheese on one half of the omelette. Fold the other half onto the cheese.

5. Leave in the pan for another 2 minutes, then let the cooked omelette slide onto a plate.
6. Fill the inside of the omelette with lettuce leaves if preferred. Serve immediately while still crispy and warm.

Zucchini Taco Bites

Nutritional Facts Per Serving	
Calories	504
Fat	41.14g
Net Carb	5.21 g
Total Carbs:	9.61 g
Fiber:	4.4 g
Protein	24.69 g

Prep Time: *5 minutes/* ***Cook Time: 1*** *5/* ***Servings:*** *2*

Ingredients

- 120 g zucchini cut in 3 mm slices, approx. ½ medium zucchini
- 1 tsp ghee or another type of cooking oil
- ¼ medium onion
- 200 g ground beef
- 40 g cheddar cheese, grated
- 3 tbsp sour cream
- ½ avocado
- 1 tsp taco seasoning
- Pepper and salt, to taste

Instructions

1. While preheating the oven at 392°F, cut the zucchini into thin slices, about 3 mm thick.
2. Heat the ghee in a pan then sauté the onion in for 2 minutes. Gently throw in the ground beef with the taco seasoning. Cook for 3 more minutes.
3. Put a scant tablespoonful of the cooked beef on the zucchini slices. Place in the oven to bake for 7 minutes.
4. Add the grated cheddar cheese on top and rebake for an additional 3 minutes.
5. Top with some sour cream and a piece of avocado.
6. Serve and enjoy!

Grilled Beef Steak

Nutritional Facts Per Serving	
Calories	568
Fat	48.5g
Net Carb	0.5 g
Total Carbs:	1 g
Fiber:	0.5 g
Protein	30.6 g

Prep Time: 20 minutes/ **Cook Time:** 7 / *Servings:* 4

Ingredients

- 4 pcs ribeye steak 1 ½ inch thick, boneless
- 3 tbsp dijon mustard
- 2 tbsp lemon juice, freshly squeezed
- 3 tbsp olive oil
- 1 tsp salt
- ½ tsp black pepper, freshly ground

Instructions

1. Take out the steak from the fridge 20 minutes prior to grilling. Allow cooling at room temperature in a covered container.
2. While preheating the grill to high, combine the rest of the ingredients together in a bowl.
3. Coat both sides of the steak with the mixture. Grill the meat for 4-5 minutes. When one side is slightly charred, flip the steak and grill for another 3-4 minutes to make a medium-rare steak.
4. Transfer to a cutting board and let stand for 5 minutes to cool.
5. Slice into slivers and serve with any low-carb veggies or salad of your choice.

Keto Deviled Eggs

Nutritional Facts Per Serving	
Calories	264
Fat	23.9g
Net Carb	0.9 g
Total Carbs:	1.1 g
Fiber:	0.2 g
Protein	11.3 g

Prep Time: *5 minutes/* **Cook Time:** *6/* **Servings:** *2*

Ingredients

- 4 eggs, medium-sized
- 1 tsp dijon mustard
- 3 tbsp mayonnaise, low-carb
- 1/4 tsp paprika
- 1/4 tsp cayenne pepper
- Salt, to taste
- Ground black pepper, to taste

Instructions

1. Hard boil the eggs for 6-7 minutes.
2. Drain the water, then peel off the shells of the eggs. Slice lengthwise to produce two halves.
3. Scoop out the yolks from the halved eggs and transfer these to a bowl. Mash the yolks together with dijon mustard, mayonnaise, cayenne pepper, and enough salt for flavor. Mix well with a fork.
4. Fill the egg whites with the mashed yolks. Garnish with ground black pepper and paprika on top.
5. Serve and enjoy!

Broccoli and Shrimp Sautéed in Butter

Nutritional Facts Per Serving	
Calories	277
Fat	14.28
Net Carb	3.42 g
Total Carbs:	4.62 g
Fiber:	1.2 g
Protein	31.88 g

Prep Time: 5 minutes/ *Cook Time:* 7/ *Servings:* 2

Ingredients

- 1 cup broccoli, cut into small pieces
- 1 clove garlic, crushed
- 300 g shrimp, cleaned
- 2 tbsp butter
- 1 tsp lemon juice
- Salt, to taste

Instructions

1. Chop the broccoli into small portions or whichever size you prefer, but smaller pieces cook faster.
2. Melt the butter in a preheated pan. Gently toss in the chopped broccoli and crushed garlic when the butter becomes hot (but not smoking). Stir to cook.
3. Leave over the heat for 3-4 minutes. Stir from time to time.
4. Clean the shrimp before adding them to the pan. Let it cook for around 3-4 minutes.
5. Once the shrimp turns pink and opaque, drizzle the lemon juice all over.
6. Transfer to a plate and serve.

Fat Head Pizza

Nutritional Facts Per Serving	
Calories	117
Fat	9.1
Net Carb	1.2 g
Total Carbs:	1.6 g
Fiber:	0.4 g
Protein	7.6 g

Prep Time: *10 minutes/* **Cook Time:** *20/* **Servings:** *8*

Ingredients

Fathead Pizza Crust:

- 1.5 cup shredded mozzarella
- 2 oz cream cheese
- 1/3 cup coconut flour
- 2 eggs
- 1 tsp dried oregano (optional)
- 1 tsp flaxseed meal (optional)

Suggested Topping:

- 10 leaves fresh basil
- 4 slices salami
- 1 3/4 oz Bocconcini (1 ball)
- 5 g pepperoni
- 3 tbsp marinara sauce, any low-carb tomato sauce you choose
- 1/2 cup mozzarella, shredded

Instructions

1. Preheat oven to 400°F.
2. Microwave the cream cheese and mozzarella in a bowl together. Begin with 50 seconds, then stir the mixture occasionally so as not to burn it. Replace in the microwave and repeat until fully melted.
3. Combine the spices in the melted cheese. Lessen the amount of salt you add since the other ingredients already contain enough

salt. Ideally, skip adding the salt in the mixture.

4. Crack the eggs into the cheese as well. Fold altogether with a spoon or a spatula to combine.

5. Throw in the coconut flour into the mixture. Knead to consistency. If you knead too much, the dough will harden and you may have to replace it in the microwave to warm it up.

6. Prepare a pan or pizza pan layered with parchment paper. Cover the entire surface of the pan with the dough. Spread it with your hands and push holes in the dough with a fork to prevent the formation of bubbles.

7. Make sure the oven is preheated at 400°F before baking the pizza in it for 12-15 minutes until brown. Baking time depends upon the thickness and size of the dough.

8. Observe the dough carefully since it bakes faster than regular crust. Burst out any bubbles that form.

9. When the dough is cooked enough, spread the tomato sauce and your favorite toppings on the surface. Bake again for 5 minutes to cook the toppings.

10. Transfer to a flat plate and enjoy. Slice with a sharp knife or pizza cutter to make 8 triangles. Best enjoyed with loved ones.

Keto Bread with Almond and Coconut Flour

Nutritional Facts Per Serving	
Calories	475
Fat	38.16
Net Carb	5.82 g
Total Carbs:	17.02 g
Fiber:	11.2 g
Protein	19.22 g

Prep Time: *10 minutes/* **Cook Time:** *30/* **Servings:** *4*

Ingredients

- 1 1/2 cup almond flour
- 5 tbsp coconut flour
- 1 1/2 tbsp psyllium husk powder
- 2 tbsp ground flaxseed
- 1 tsp baking soda
- 6 eggs
- 1 tbsp coconut oil liquid
- 1 tbsp butter, melted

Instructions

1. Get all the ingredients ready for the journey!
2. Preheat oven to 200 °C; put the eggs in a big bowl and mix well for 3-4 minutes.
3. Add the butter and coconut oil and mix again for a minute.
4. Add the almond flour, coconut flour, baking soda, psyllium husk, and ground flaxseed to the mixture and mix again. Let the mixture sit for about 15 minutes.
5. Spread a little bit of coconut oil in a loaf pan so that the bread doesn't stick and put the mixture in it.
6. Bake for 25 minutes and check with a toothpick to see if it's fully cooked – stick the toothpick in it, if it comes out clean, it's ready.
7. Let it cool down for 5 minutes.

Easy Cloud Buns

Nutritional Facts Per Serving	
Calories	50
Fat	4.5
Net Carb	0.5 g
Total Carbs:	0.5 g
Fiber:	0 g
Protein	2.5 g

Prep Time: 10 minutes/ **Cook Time:** 30/ *Servings:* 10

Ingredients

- 3 large eggs, separated
- 1/8 teaspoon cream of tartar
- 3 ounces cream cheese, chopped

Instructions

1. Preheat the oven to 300°F and line a baking sheet with parchment.
2. Beat the egg whites until foamy then beat in the cream of tartar until the whites are shiny and opaque with soft peaks.
3. In a separate bowl, beat the cream cheese and egg yolks until well combined then fold in the egg white mixture.
4. Spoon the batter onto the baking sheet in ¼-cup circles about 2 inches apart.
5. Bake for 30 minutes until the buns are firm to the touch.

Chicken Breast with Eggplant, Zucchini and Spinach

Nutritional Facts Per Serving	
Calories	369
Fat	20.4
Net Carb	8.54 g
Total Carbs:	13.84 g
Fiber:	5.3 g
Protein	35.06 g

Prep Time: 5 minutes/ Cook Time: 20/ Servings: 3

Ingredients

- 400 g chicken breast, skinless
- 1 medium zucchini diced, unpeeled
- ½ medium eggplant diced, unpeeled
- 2 cups spinach, cut in pieces
- 150 g mushrooms, sliced
- 1 clove garlic, minced
- 1/3 medium onion chopped in small pieces or sliced
- 1 tbsp ghee

For the marinade (optional):

- 3 tbsp extra virgin olive oil
- 1/5 cup lemon juice
- 2 cloves garlic, minced
- 1/4 tsp salt
- 1 tsp black pepper

Instructions

1. If you like to marinate the chicken, combine the ingredients for the marinade together in a bowl. Stir well.
2. Dice the chicken. Place in a bag or plastic box along with the marinade. Leave in the fridge for 3 hours.
3. Heat a tablespoon of ghee in a large pan. Sauté the minced garlic and onion in the oil for 2-3 minutes. Stir occasionally.

4. Slice the eggplant into cubes and toss these into the pan. Cook for another 2-3 minutes.

5. Cut the mushroom into slices and then dice the zucchini. Add them into the pan as well. Leave to cook. This may take an additional 2-3 minutes.

6. Stir the chicken into the vegetable mixture for 6-7 minutes to cook thoroughly.

7. Put the spinach in and leave for 5 minutes more. When the leaves wilt, remove from the heat.

8. Serve in a bowl and enjoy.

Scrambled Eggs with Mushrooms and Cottage Cheese

Nutritional Facts Per Serving	
Calories	210
Fat	18.8
Net Carb	2.5 g
Total Carbs:	3 g
Fiber:	0.5 g
Protein	9 g

Prep Time: *10 minutes/* **Cook Time:** *10/* **Servings:** *3*

Ingredients

- 3 eggs
- 1 cup button mushrooms, rinsed and sliced
- 1/2 medium-sized onion, finely chopped
- 3 tbsp olive oil
- 1/4 tsp oregano
- 1/4 cup cottage cheese
- 1/2 tsp sea salt
- 1/4 tsp black pepper

Instructions

1. Place a large skillet over medium-high heat. Let the olive oil heat in the pan. Sauté the finely chopped onions in the oil until they become translucent. Drop in the sliced mushrooms and let it simmer until the liquid in the pan evaporates. Stir well with oregano, pepper, and salt. Put aside.
2. Beat the eggs in a bowl. Flavor with a dash of salt and pepper enough to taste. Fry in the skillet and fold with a wooden spoon for a minute until slightly underdone.
3. Transfer to a serving plate with the mushrooms and a quarter cup of cottage cheese. Enjoy!

Low-Carb Tortillas with Ground Beef

Nutritional Facts Per Serving	
Calories	492
Fat	32.92
Net Carb	6.33 g
Total Carbs:	14,43 g
Fiber:	8.1 g
Protein	32,21 g

*Prep Time: 10 minutes/ **Cook Time:** 40/ **Servings:** 3*
Ingredients

For the tortillas:
- 3 medium eggs
- 2 egg whites
- ½ cup water
- 6 tbsp coconut flour
- 1 tbsp ground flaxseed
- ¼ tsp baking powder
- ¼ tsp paprika powder
- ¼ tsp cayenne pepper
- 1 tbsp butter

For the filling:
- 250 g ground beef
- 1/4 medium onion, diced
- 1/4 tsp cumin powder
- 1/2 tsp paprika powder
- 1/4 tsp ground oregano
- 1/4 tsp cayenne pepper
- 1/2 avocado, cut in pieces
- 1 medium tomato, cut in pieces
- 2 tbsp sour cream

Instructions

1. Start preparing the tortillas. Combine the tortilla ingredients (except the butter) in a bowl. Fold together until incorporated.
2. Melt the butter on a preheated pan, then fry the tortillas. Make the tortillas as thin as possible by turning around the pan and spreading the batter evenly.
3. Make the filling for the tortillas. Sauté the minced onion in cooking oil then brown the ground beef in the oil as well. Leave for 10 minutes to cook.
4. Season the beef with the spices and stir for 2 more minutes for the beef to fully absorb the flavors.
5. Fill the tortillas with the beef. Plop in the avocado, tomato, and sour cream in the tortilla as well. Serve and enjoy.

Grilled Stuffed Zucchini with Bacon

Nutritional Facts Per Serving	
Calories	492
Fat	32.92
Net Carb	6.33 g
Total Carbs:	14,43 g
Fiber:	8.1 g
Protein	32,21 g

Prep Time: *10 minutes/* **Cook Time:** *40/* **Servings:** *4*

Ingredients

- 4 medium-sized zucchini
- 5 tsp olive oil
- 200 g bacon
- 2 clove garlic, minced
- 1/2 onion medium-sized, chopped
- 1 tbsp spring onion, finely chopped (optional)
- 1 cup cheddar cheese, shredded
- Salt and pepper, to taste

Instructions

1. Half the zucchini lengthwise. Empty the insides by scooping out the pulp.
2. Coat the zucchini with 2 tsp of oil. Put aside for later. Chop the bacon and the pulp into small bits. Heat the remaining oil in a large skillet before sautéing the onion, garlic, pulp, and bacon. Pepper to taste.
3. Stir for about 2 minutes to cook or wait till golden brown. Remove the pan from the heat.
4. Add spoonfuls of the cooked mixture into the empty zucchini shells.
5. Top with chopped spring onion and shredded cheddar cheese.
6. Set the zucchinis over medium heat. Grill covered for around 8-10 minutes until the zucchini is tender to your liking.

7. Transfer to a plate and enjoy.

Vegetable Tart

Nutritional Facts Per Serving	
Calories	250
Fat	22
Net Carb	4.2 g
Total Carbs:	5,4 g
Fiber:	1.2 g
Protein	9.4 g

Prep Time: *10 minutes/* **Cook Time:** *1 hour/* **Servings:** *8*

Ingredients

- 6 eggs
- ½ cup heavy cream
- 8 oz cream cheese
- ½ cup shredded cheese
- ½ cup almond milk (or coconut milk)
- 12 oz zucchini
- 4 oz cauliflower
- 2 oz broccoli
- 8 oz red pepper
- 3 oz jalapeno
- 3 oz onion
- 3 cloves garlic
- Seasoning of your choice

Instructions

1. Mince the cauliflower, broccoli, garlic, onion, red pepper, and jalapeño into small cubes. Dice the zucchini as well.
2. Sauté the diced vegetables in a heated oil on a large skillet. Remove from the heat when they become soft enough but not mushy.

3. Crack the eggs in another bowl. Combine the almond milk, softened cream cheese, and heavy cream in the bowl. Mix everything to combine well.
4. Mix the vegetables into the cream cheese bowl. Stir with the cheese and seasonings of choice. Fold together until uniform.
5. Lay a foil on the base of the springform you will use to avoid seeping the mixture through the bottom. Cover with parchment paper and brush some oil on the sides and on the base. Pour the batter into the form. Bake for one hour or up till the surface of the tart is golden brown in color. The oven must be preheated to 350°F.
6. Generously dust with cheese on top after baking. Slice into wedges and serve.

Coconut Flour Pizza Bites

Nutritional Facts Per Serving	
Calories	418
Fat	31.36
Net Carb	5.98 g
Total Carbs:	12,68 g
Fiber:	6.7 g
Protein	21.2 g

Prep Time: 15 minutes/ **Cook Time:** 20 minutes/ **Servings:** 4

Ingredients

For the crust:
- 4 tbsp coconut flour
- 2 tbsp olive oil
- 1 tbsp flaxseed, ground
- 2 large eggs
- 30 g Parmesan, grated

For the topping:
- 60 g zucchini, thinly sliced
- 1/3 medium tomato sliced and cut into small pieces
- 50 g mozzarella cheese, grated
- 2 button mushrooms

Instructions

1. Preheat the oven at 392°F.
2. Put the coconut flour, olive oil, flaxseed, and Parmesan in a large bowl and whisk the eggs.
3. Mix everything together.
4. Make individual pizza patties of about 4 cm in diameter and place them in an adapted container (greased in advance). You'll have enough dough for approx. 9 to 11 patties. .

5. Cook them for about 15 minutes or until slightly brown.
6. Slice the tomatoes, zucchini, and mushrooms and quickly sauté the zucchini and the mushrooms.
7. Put the zucchini, mushrooms, and mozzarella on top of the pizza bites and bake for another 5 minutes.
8. Put the tomato slices on top of each bite and cook for another minute or two. Enjoy!

Zucchini Noodles with Meatballs

Nutritional Facts Per Serving	
Calories	575
Fat	35 g
Net Carb	4 g
Protein	52 g

*Prep Time: 10 minutes/ **Cook Time:** 20 minutes/ **Servings:** 2*

Ingredients

- 16 oz ground beef
- 200 g zucchini
- ¼ cup Parmesan
- 1 large egg, beaten
- ½ cup marinara sauce

Instructions

1. Place the beef and Parmesan cheese in a bowl. Crack the egg in the bowl as well. Knead until well combined. Flavor with your favorite seasonings. Mold into about one-inch spheres.
2. Set a pan over high heat and sear the balls in. Make sure that all sides are cooked. Lower the flame and place the lid over the pan. Leave to cook for 5 more minutes. Pour the marinara sauce and cook for another 5 minutes.
3. Use a spiralizer to make zucchini spirals.
4. Lightly oil a pan and place the zucchini in for 2 minutes. Toss to cook.
5. Transfer the noodles on a dish and serve with the meatballs on top.

WEEK 5

THIS WEEK'S MEAL PLAN

	Breakfast	Lunch	Dinner
DAY 29	Zucchini Breakfast Muffins	Crustless Keto Quiche/ Frittata	Beef and Eggplant Keto Kebab
DAY 30	Cauliflower Hash Browns	Greek Keto Salad	Low-Carb Taco Bake

RECIPES FOR WEEK 5

<u>Zucchini Breakfast Muffins</u>

Nutritional Facts Per Serving	
Calories	185
Fat	16 g
Net Carb	1.5 g
Total Carbs:	1,9 g
Fiber:	0.4 g
Protein	8.7 g

Prep Time: *15 minutes/* ***Cook Time:*** *20 minutes/* ***Servings:*** *1 2*

Ingredients

- 6 eggs
- 1 zucchini, medium-sized
- 5 slices bacon
- 2 tbsp sour cream
- 1 cup heavy cream
- 1 cup shredded cheddar cheese
- 1 tbsp mayonnaise
- 1 tbsp mustard
- 1/2 cup coconut milk
- 1 oz dill
- 1 jalapeno small size
- 4 oz red pepper
- Salt and pepper, to taste

Instructions

1. Shred your zucchini into thin pieces and dust with some salt. Put aside for a few minutes to release the moisture.

2. Chop the dill into fine pieces, then mince your jalapeno and red pepper.
3. Crispy fry the bacon slices for around 5 minutes or simply heat them in the microwave. Cut into bits.
4. Strain all the unnecessary liquids from the grated zucchini. Press it with your hands to squeeze out the extracts. Alternatively, use a cheesecloth to do this. Transfer all of the chopped vegetables in a bowl and toss to mix well. Add in the cheese and bacon bits.
5. Crack the eggs in a separate bowl. Blend together with the sour cream, mustard, heavy cream, and mayo. Include the coconut milk as well. Adjust the flavor with salt and pepper.
6. Transfer the vegetable mix into 12 muffin forms. Distribute evenly. Gently add in the egg mixture into the cups. Remember to fill only ⅔ of the cup. Combine the two mixture with a spoon. Stir well.
7. Bake in the oven preheated at 370°F for 20-25 minutes. Make sure the muffins are golden and firm before removing from the oven.
8. Unmold from the cups and serve on a plate.

Crustless Keto Quiche/Frittata

Nutritional Facts Per Serving	
Calories	392
Fat	29,46 g
Net Carb	5.36 g
Total Carbs:	6,66g
Fiber:	1.3 g
Protein	25.63 g

Prep Time: 10 minutes/ **Cook Time:** 35 minutes/ *Servings: 4*

Ingredients

- 6 large eggs
- 100 g feta cheese, crumbled
- 60 g gouda cheese, grated
- 30 g Parmesan cheese, grated
- 50 g heavy cream
- ½ onion, diced
- 100 g mushrooms, sliced
- 60 g baby spinach cut into small pieces
- 100 g ham cut into small pieces
- 1 tbsp coconut oil
- 1/8 tsp salt (1 dash of salt)

Instructions

1. Pre-heat oven at 392°F.
2. Whisk the eggs in a large bowl.
3. Add spinach, mushrooms, onion, feta, gouda, Parmesan, ham, cream, and salt and mix everything well.
4. Grease the pie plate with oil – make sure to spread it on the walls as well, so that the quiche doesn't stick.
5. Pour the mixture into the pie plate, spread it well and bake for 35 minutes at 392°F.
6. Let it cool for a couple of minutes.

7. Enjoy!

Beef and Eggplant Keto Kebab

Nutritional Facts Per Serving	
Calories	*444*
Fat	*30,2 g*
Net Carb	*3.1 g*
Total Carbs:	*6 g*
Fiber:	*2.9 g*
Protein	*37.5 g*

Prep Time: *20 minutes/* ***Cook Time:*** *20 minutes/* ***Servings:*** *3*

Ingredients

- ½ large eggplant
- 1 lb lean ground beef, grass-fed
- 2 free-range eggs, beaten
- 1 cup parsley leaves, finely chopped
- 4 garlic cloves, crushed
- ¼ cup olive oil
- ½ tsp chili pepper, freshly ground
- 1 tsp salt
- ½ tsp black pepper, freshly ground
- 1 tsp oregano
- ½ tsp dried thyme
- 3 tbsp oil for the grill pan
- Wooden skewers soaked in water

Instructions

1. Slice eggplants in a circular shape (about half-inch thick).
2. Generously sprinkle with salt and set aside for 10 minutes to remove the bitterness.
3. In a large bowl, combine the meat with parsley, onions, garlic, olive oil, chili pepper, salt, black pepper, oregano, thyme, and eggs. Mix well with your hands and form patties to fit eggplant slices.

4. Preheat a large, non-stick grill pan over medium-high heat and lightly brush with oil.
5. Rinse eggplant slices and gently press with your hands to squeeze the excess water.
6. Thread eggplant slices and meatballs onto soaked skewers and place on the preheated grill pan.
7. Cook for 15 minutes, gently turning a couple of times.

Cauliflower Hash Browns

Nutritional Facts Per Serving	
Calories	*88*
Fat	*7,2 g*
Net Carb	*1.9 g*
Total Carbs:	*3.3 g*
Fiber:	*1.4 g*
Protein	*3.5 g*

*Prep Time: 10 minutes/ **Cook Time:** 20 minutes/ **Servings:** 6*

Ingredients

- 1 cauliflower (small head, raw)
- 2 large eggs
- 2 tbsp coconut oil for frying
- 1/2 tsp onion powder
- 1/4 tsp garlic powder
- 2 tbsp almond flour
- 2 tbsp green onions
- 1/4 tsp kosher salt
- 1/8 tsp black pepper

Instructions

1. Rinse the cauliflower thoroughly with water. Dry completely. Discard the leaves and chop into little portions.
2. Transfer the chopped cauliflower in a food processor and pulse until you get rice-size pieces.
3. Pour the cauliflower rice in a heat-safe bowl and leave in the microwave for a minute, enough to make the rice soft.
4. Place all the remaining ingredients in a bowl. Mix in the cauliflower. Blend with a spoon until the mixture is uniform.
5. Set a non-stick skillet over medium-high heat. Heat the coconut oil in the pan and gently pour the mixture in.
6. Fry for around 4-5 minutes. Use a turner flipper to turn the hash browns over gently.

7. Remove from the heat once cooked then serve in a plate.
8. Enjoy warm or at room temperature.

Greek Keto Salad

Nutritional Facts Per Serving	
Calories	266
Fat	22,89 g
Net Carb	8.09 g
Total Carbs:	10.79 g
Fiber:	2.7 g
Protein	6.76 g

Prep Time: 30 minutes/ *Servings:* 4

Ingredients

For salad:

- 4 medium tomatoes, chopped
- ½ cucumber, diced
- 140 g feta cheese, crumbled
- ½ medium red onion, sliced
- 1 small green bell pepper, diced
- 12 olives

For dressing:

- ½ tsp dried oregano
- 4 tbsp extra virgin olive oil
- 1 tbsp red wine vinegar
- ½ garlic clove, minced
- Salt

Instructions

1. Cut the tomatoes, cucumber, onion, feta, bell pepper.
2. Put them in a salad bowl together with the olives.
3. Mix everything together and add the salt and the oregano.
4. Whisk together the olive oil, vinegar and the minced garlic clove in a separate cup. Enjoy it with someone you love!

Low-Carb Taco Bake

Nutritional Facts Per Serving	
Calories	*541*
Fat	*43,4 g*
Net Carb	*6 g*
Total Carbs:	*7.4 g*
Fiber:	*1.4 g*
Protein	*30.8 g*

Prep Time: 15 minutes/ *Cook Time:* 1 hour/ *Servings:* 4

Ingredients

For crust:

- 2 eggs
- 2 oz cream cheese
- 1/3 cup heavy cream
- 1/2 tsp taco seasoning
- 4 oz cheddar cheese, shredded
- 1 tsp olive oil for greasing

For topping:

- 1/2 lb ground beef
- 1 tbsp olive oil
- 1/4 cup tomato paste
- 4 oz cheddar cheese, shredded
- 1-2 tsp taco seasoning (up to your liking)
- 3 oz green bell pepper, chopped
- 1 tbsp onion, chopped
- Salt and pepper, to taste

Other extra toppings (optional):

- 2 tbsp sour cream
- 1 medium jalapeno (sliced, for spiciness)
- 1 oz mozzarella cheese (for extra cheesy texture)

Instructions

Making the crust:

1. Crack the eggs in a bowl and beat together with the cream cheese until you obtain a smooth texture. Include the seasonings and heavy cream in the mix as well.
2. Prep the baking dish you will use by greasing it well. Place the shredded cheddar cheese on the base of the dish. Spread the egg mixture all over the dish evenly.
3. Take the dish to the oven and allow to bake for 25-30 minutes at 375°F. After baking, leave for 5 more minutes to cool.

Prepare the topping:

4. In a pan over medium high heat, fry the ground beef with olive oil until brown. You can add onion, salt, and pepper for taste.
5. Once the beef is cooked, strain the fat if you prefer a drier final dish. Pour the tomato sauce into the pan of beef. Throw in the seasonings and green bell pepper.
6. Pour the topping on the surface of the crust. Sprinkle a generous amount of cheese as well. You can add some jalapeno slices for spiciness (optional). You can even add more cheese if you want it even more cheesy.
7. Set the oven to 350°F. Leave in the oven for an additional 20 minutes. Wait until the cheese is nice and bubbly.
8. Top with some sour cream (optional) and serve with your favorite low-carb salad.

CONCLUSION

Falling off the horse happens to everyone. What happens next depends on how fat-adapted you are. In the beginning, before you've gone two or three weeks without carbs, you may be starting over at square one. Some people never get fat-adapted because they don't have the patience to go carb-free for three to eight weeks. I'm not talking about willpower. Keto is easy if you can stay focused. I half-heartedly did keto for years, going low carb for a few days, then binging for a couple weeks, and repeating the cycle. It made me sicker than I was before.

Let's say you've been doing keto for a couple of weeks and you decide for whatever reason to eat a slice of pizza. The carbs are going to immediately trigger cravings for more carbs. You'll start eating anything with carbs: crackers, cookies, etc…it just happens. You have no control over it. Your body wants carbs, and it takes over. Sound familiar? If you do this, it could take you a week or two of no carbs to get back to where you were. Your weight will come back, and those two weeks will be wasted.

However, once you're fat-adapted and you do the same thing, starting with a slice of pizza and escalating to an entire pint of ice cream, then you will wake up in the morning and most likely NOT have carb cravings. Actually, I can only attest to MY experiences here. That's what happened to me. I didn't have carb cravings, but the weight still came back on. It took me a week to get back to my previous weight—after one day. We're talking ten pounds in one day! However, the lack of carb cravings made it EASIER for me to get right back up on the horse and continue on.

So, rather than worrying about the next time you can have your favorite food with carbs, focus on how good eating keto makes you feel. In our now-closed Facebook group, Kassie Ewers famously said, "Every time I see someone eating fries or something else I can't eat, I look down and wiggle my toes and think, 'Yeah. Toes are better than fries.'" The real goal is to not die of diabetes, renal failure, heart attack, stroke, hypertension, fatty liver, dementia, Alzheimer's, or cancer. Those are the real goals. Weight loss and fitness are natural side effects of good health. Stay motivated! Peruse the ketogenic forums. Spread the word about how you have lost weight and reclaimed your health. Save someone else's life! These things will make you so much happier than a pint of ice cream, especially when you can make yourself some keto mousse or ice cream and be completely happy with it!

CPSIA information can be obtained
at www.ICGtesting.com
Printed in the USA
LVHW061056090621
689781LV00003B/303